Fashions in
Godey's Lady's Book
1837–69

With little competition and the support of loyal subscribers, *Godey's Lady's Book* enjoyed immense popularity shortly after its inception in 1830 and went on to become an institution and a leading fashion oracle until the late 1860s, when other periodicals began to make inroads into the *Godey's* readership. Although these publications were, in the main, clones of *Godey's*, they offered subscribers choice and variety.

When the magazine was first launched by Louis B. Godey in July 1830, it focused on short stories, serials and essays (pirated from English publications) which he assumed would be of interest to ladies. Sentimentally romantic, the contents had little depth or substance, or any specific reference to fashions. *Godey's* had published its first fashion plate in 1830, but it was without any description or commentary. For a few years following, fashion illustrations appeared sporadically. The initial plates—with little regard for copyright ethics—were reproductions of ones that had appeared earlier in French and English periodicals. In January 1837, Sarah Josepha Hale (1788–1879) took charge as editor and, in short order, the magazine began to reflect her input. Her creed was to make her work "national . . . American . . . and a miscellany which although devoted to general literature is more expressly designed to mark the progress of female improvement."

By any standards in any period, Mrs. Hale was a remarkable woman. In her day, her achievements were nothing short of phenomenal. A nearly penniless widow with five young children and no particular training, she not only carved out a highly successful career as a magazine editor at a time when it was virtually impossible for women to support themselves, but even earned a place in history. An ardent feminist and a zealous activist in causes in which she believed, Mrs. Hale is credited with initiating the movement to make Thanksgiving a national holiday, helping to organize Vassar College, the first collegiate institution for women, and working for the completion of the Bunker Hill monument and for the preservation of Mount Vernon. Using her column, "Editor's Table," she championed women's causes and spoke out against a variety of social injustices. All this she somehow accomplished with the demeanor of a proper Victorian lady.

Shortly after she took over as editor, Mrs. Hale began to hire local artists to redraw for *Godey's* the fashions that appeared in foreign publications. As a result, a single illustration may be a composite of sources as well as of dates, some as much as a year apart. While these colored fashion plates served to inform the subscribers of the latest fashions, many of the gowns, particularly those for evening, were hardly appropriate for the lifestyle of most of *Godey's* readers, and one wonders if Mrs. Hale or anyone on her staff really ever came face to face with many of the fashions they featured in the colored plates. The captions were often vague as to the fabrics used in the dresses, and at times the colors as described in the text do not correspond with those in the hand-painted plates. In spite of these shortcomings and the impracticality of some of the high styles shown, these plates did supply the stuff of dreams for many an American woman.

Reading between the lines, one can detect that fashions were not high on Mrs. Hale's priority list. She informs her readers that questions relating to fashion were not to be addressed to her; they were to be sent to someone called "the Editress of the Fashion Department." However, she was an astute businesswoman and knew the importance of fashions to women. In due time, the magazine began to include more appropriate, simplified versions of European fashions expressed in clear black-and-white drawings. These were generally day clothes and could easily be "read" by dressmakers.

The closing years of the 1830s marked the end of the postclassical Romantic style. What ensued was a sentimental Gothic configuration. In 1837, Victoria became Queen of England. The crowning of a fragile girl in her teens as the head of a world power was a fantasy come to life. Women adulated her; they began to emulate her looks and followed her every movement with great interest. Aware of this fascination with the young queen, *Godey's* hired a correspondent, Mrs. Lydia H. Sigourney, who reported on the royal activities in London. However, brought up in a Protestant German tradition by a strict mother, Victoria shunned elaborate, opulent clothes. Following her example, fashions became nearly devoid of ornamentation. The accent was on plainness and modesty, reflecting the emphasis on female decorum. By 1840, skirt hemlines fell to the floor, totally concealing ankles and feet. Sleeves became so narrow that they restricted the movement of arms above the elbow. Rigidly boned, elongated bodices constrained the torso, giving the silhouette the static aspect of Gothic arches. Bonnets were designed to keep the wearer's eyes chastely forward, precluding flirtatious sidelong glances. Relying mainly on the fabric and a minimum of trimming to give them distinction, the fashions of the 1840s appear rather stark and lacking in excitement.

In 1852, Napoleon III and Empress Eugénie revived the French court. The fashion-conscious empress soon put an end to Victorian austerity. Frederick Worth, an Englishman who founded French couture in 1858, provided Eugénie and her friends with fabulous gowns of magnificent silks made more luxurious by a multitude of laces, ribbons, fringes, feathers and artificial flowers. To accommodate the very full, wide skirts, which could no longer be supported by layers of petticoats, inventors looked back to the Spanish farthingale and produced a wired "cage," hoopskirt or crinoline, which *Godey's* refers to as the "bustle."

Until the late 1860s, few American women could afford French gowns. While *Godey's* included some copies of French fashion plates, many of the French gowns illustrated were simplified New York or Philadelphia versions. These are probably a more accurate record of the fashions worn in America during this period. By the mid-1860s, the hoopskirt went into eclipse and narrower skirts acquired a train. For a short time, to facilitate walking, an overskirt was looped up over an ankle-length underskirt and held in place by straps or bands. Although this style was short-lived, it created a new form which, by the late 1860s, evolved into a bustle that extended the back.

The period 1837–69 saw many sociological, political, cultural and technological changes, among which were the invention of the sewing machine and the graded pattern. Both of these eventually led to mass production. Although mail-order shopping through catalogues came later in the century, *Godey's* offered a shopping service. A reader could indicate what she wanted and, for a small fee, *Godey's* would try to meet the request.

During this period undergarments became an important part of a woman's wardrobe. Until the 1830s, women wore only a simple shift under their gowns. This shift often served also as a nightdress. Plain at first, before the end of the century underwear became as elaborate as outerwear.

After the Civil War, the nature of American society began to change rapidly. Reconstruction, new technology and widening industrialization produced a growing American moneyed aristocracy and spreading urbanization. Fashion-minded ladies started to look for more sophistication in their magazines, closer to that featured in European publications. When compared to such competitors as *Peterson's* and *Graham's*, *Godey's* began to look provincial and old-fashioned. Unfortunately, Mrs. Hale, who fought so hard for women's rights to education and a measure of equality with men, did not recognize that, in post–Civil War America, women had started to make some progress on the road to "female improvement," and that their interests and range of activities had broadened accordingly.

Godey continued to publish to a shrinking readership until he sold the magazine in 1877. In December 1877, at ninety, Sarah Josepha Hale wrote her final editorial. The following year, the new owners moved the headquarters to New York. Although they continued to publish the magazine for some twenty years, they could not recapture for *Godey's Lady's Book* the unique position it had enjoyed in American society from the late 1830s to the late 1860s.

Fashions and Costumes from Godey's Lady's Book

Including 8 Plates in Full Color

Edited and with an Introduction by

Stella Blum

Director of the Kent State University Museum

Dover Publications, Inc., New York

Copyright © 1985 by Dover Publications, Inc.
All rights reserved under Pan American and International Copyright Conventions.

Published in Canada by General Publishing Company, Ltd., 30 Lesmill Road, Don Mills, Toronto, Ontario.
Published in the United Kingdom by Constable and Company, Ltd., 10 Orange Street, London WC2H 7EG.

Fashions and Costumes from Godey's Lady's Book: Including 8 Plates in Full Color is a new work, first published by Dover Publications, Inc., in 1985.

Manufactured in the United States of America
Dover Publications, Inc., 31 East 2nd Street, Mineola, N.Y. 11501

Library of Congress Cataloging in Publication Data

Main entry under title:

Fashions and costumes from Godey's lady's book.

1. Fashion—United States—History—19th century. I. Blum, Stella. II. Godey's magazine.
GT610.F37 1985   391'.2'0973   84-21208
ISBN 0-486-24841-0 (pbk.)

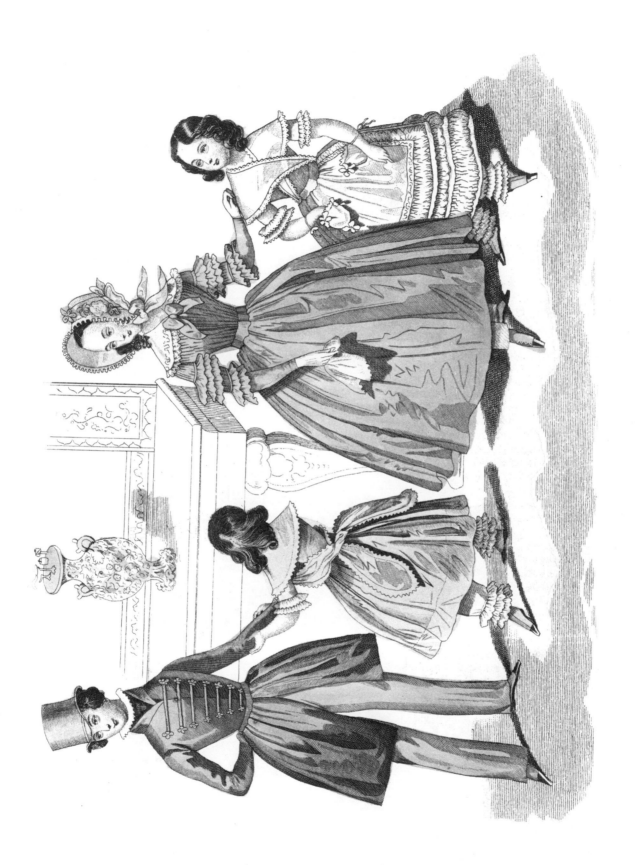

Children's fashions (10/37).

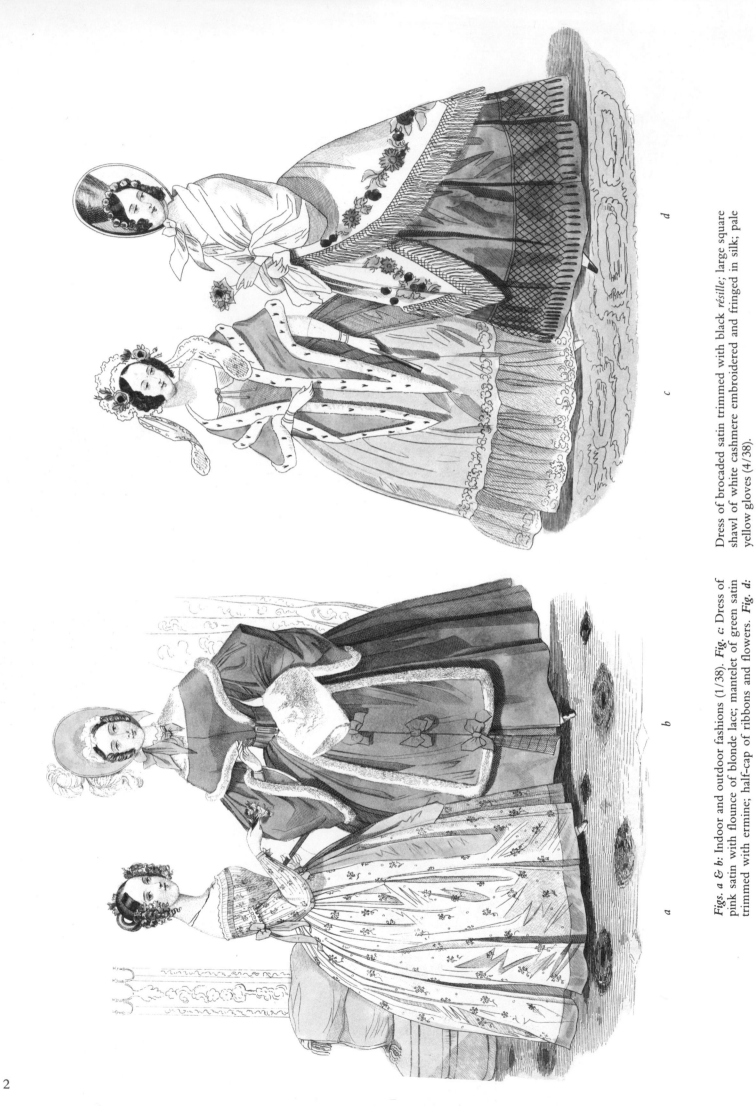

2

Figs. a & b: Indoor and outdoor fashions (1/38). *Fig. c:* Dress of pink satin with flounce of blonde lace; mantelet of green satin trimmed with ermine; half-cap of ribbons and flowers. *Fig. d:* Dress of brocaded satin trimmed with black *résille;* large square shawl of white cashmere embroidered and fringed in silk; pale yellow gloves (4/38).

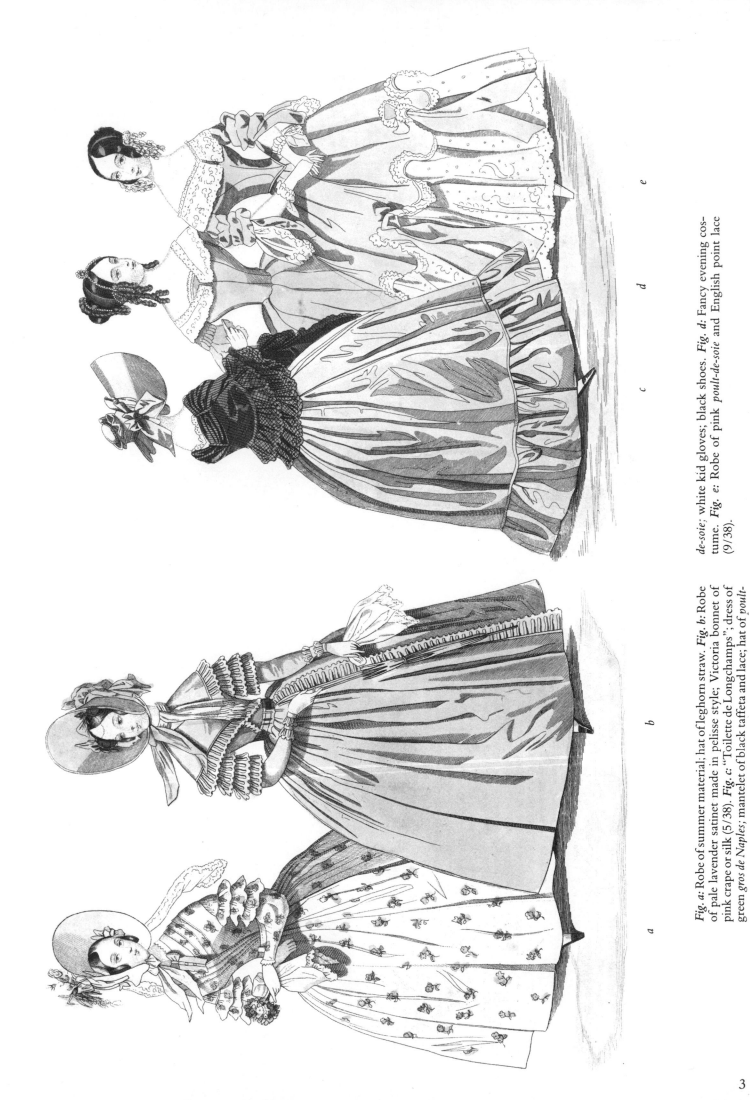

Fig. a: Robe of summer material: hat of leghorn straw. *Fig. b:* Robe of pale lavender satinet made in pelisse style; Victoria bonnet of pink crape or silk (5/38). *Fig. c:* "Toilette de Longchamps"; dress of green *gros de Naples;* mantelet of black taffeta and lace; hat of *poult-*

de-soie; white kid gloves; black shoes. *Fig. d:* Fancy evening costume. *Fig. e:* Robe of pink *poult-de-soie* and English point lace (9/38).

3

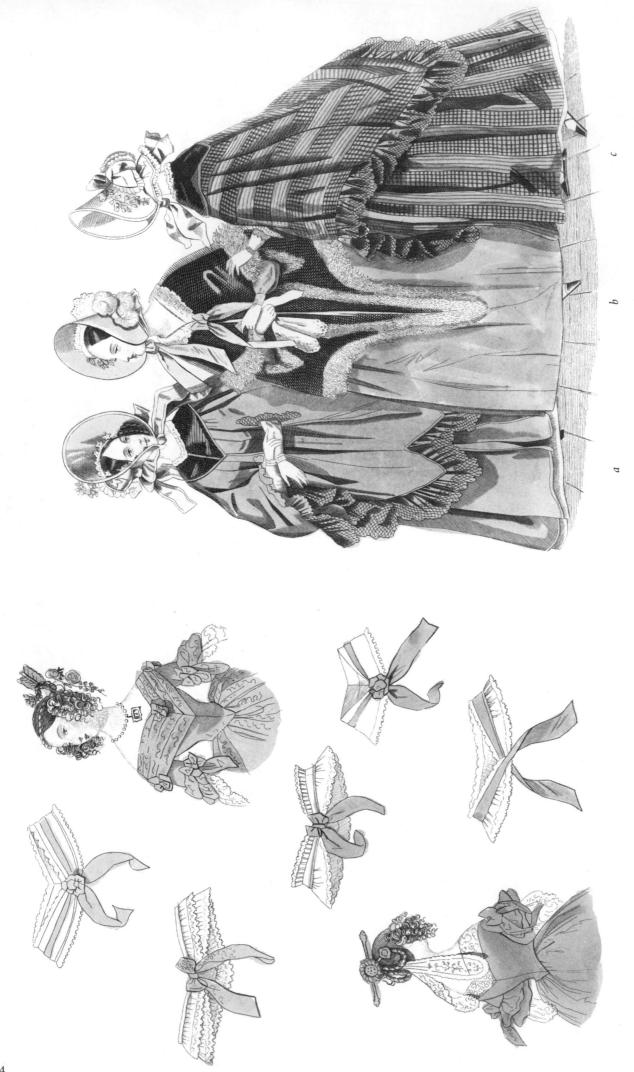

4

LEFT: Neckline and head accessories (10/38). RIGHT: *Fig. a:*
Mantle of green satin trimmed with green velvet and black lace;
bonnet of straw-colored satin. *Fig. b:* Walking or carriage costume;

dress of tan *poult-de-soie;* "Mantel chale" of black velvet trimmed
with fur; hat "capote" of pink velvet; pale yellow gloves; black
shoes. *Fig. c:* Back view of a costume similar to Fig. a. (12/38).

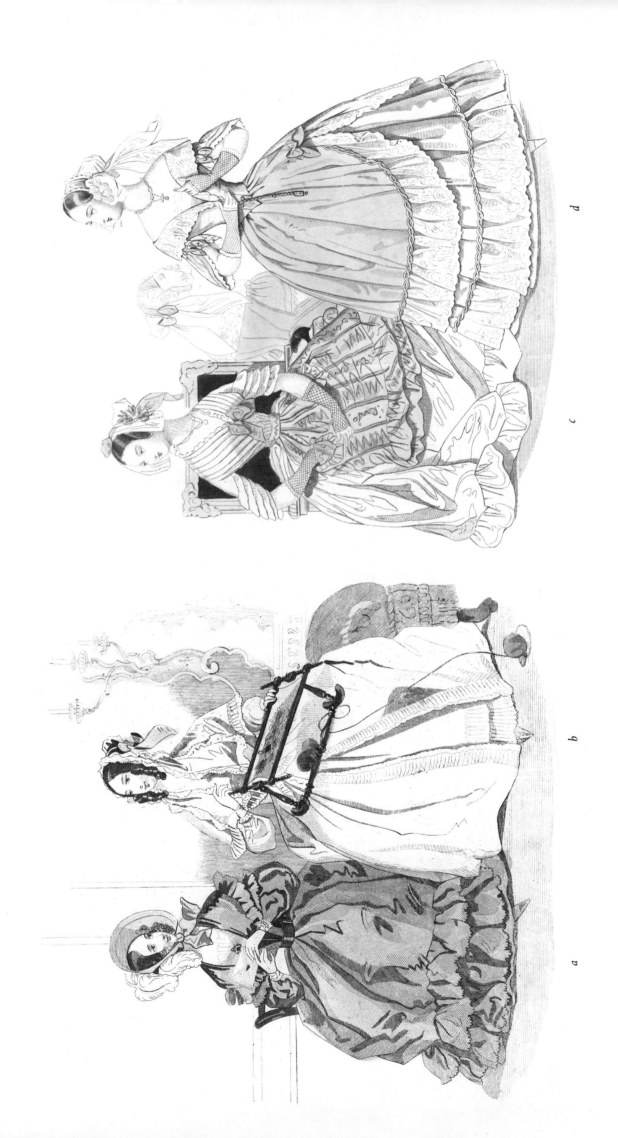

Fig. a: Dress of shot silk with bishop sleeves. *Fig. b:* Morning negligé; white cambric dress open in front to display matching underdress; cap of tulle of fine muslin (2/40). *Fig. c:* Home dress of white muslin; apron of *broché* silk; cap, "The Peasant's Cap"; half-

long black netting mittens. *Fig. d:* Dinner or evening dress of *poult-de-soie* shot with *glacé de blanc*; cap of blonde lace; black net mittens; white satin shoes (5/40).

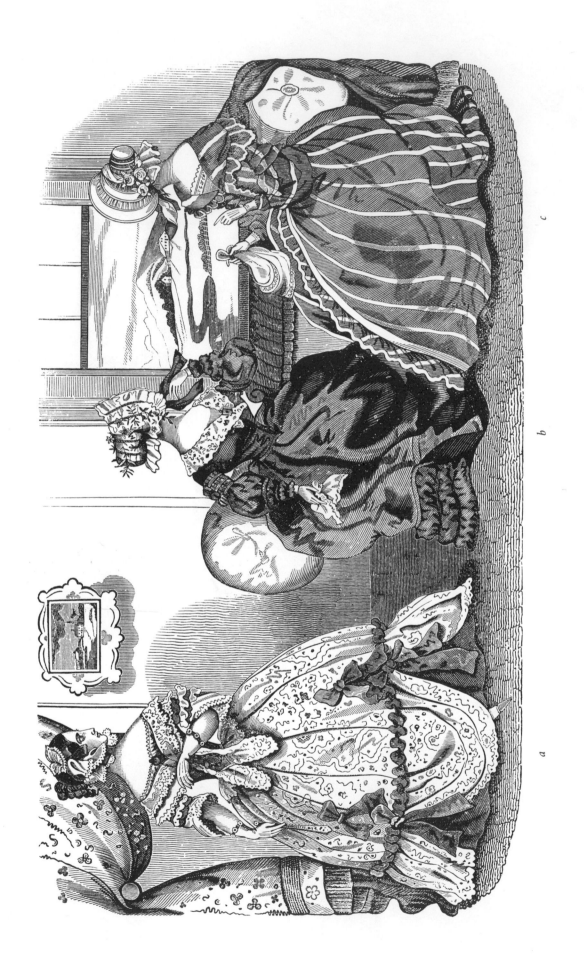

Fig. a: Evening dress of white lace over pink; headdress of lace and ribbons. *Fig. b*: "Levantine" dress; hat of white lace. *Fig. c*: Dress of striped changeable silk (5/40).

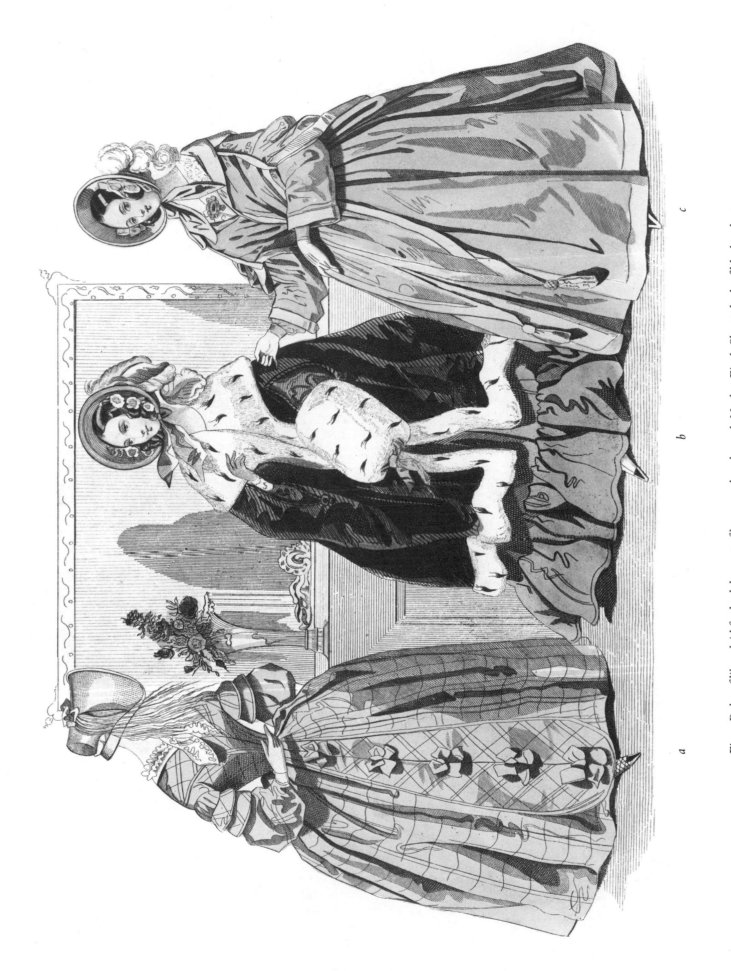

Fig. a: Robe of lilac plaid foulard; bonnet of lemon-colored *gros de Naples. Fig. b:* Short cloak of black velvet trimmed with white fur; gray silk bonnet. *Fig. c:* Manteau of brown satin, wadded and worn with cape; hat of blue satin (9/40).

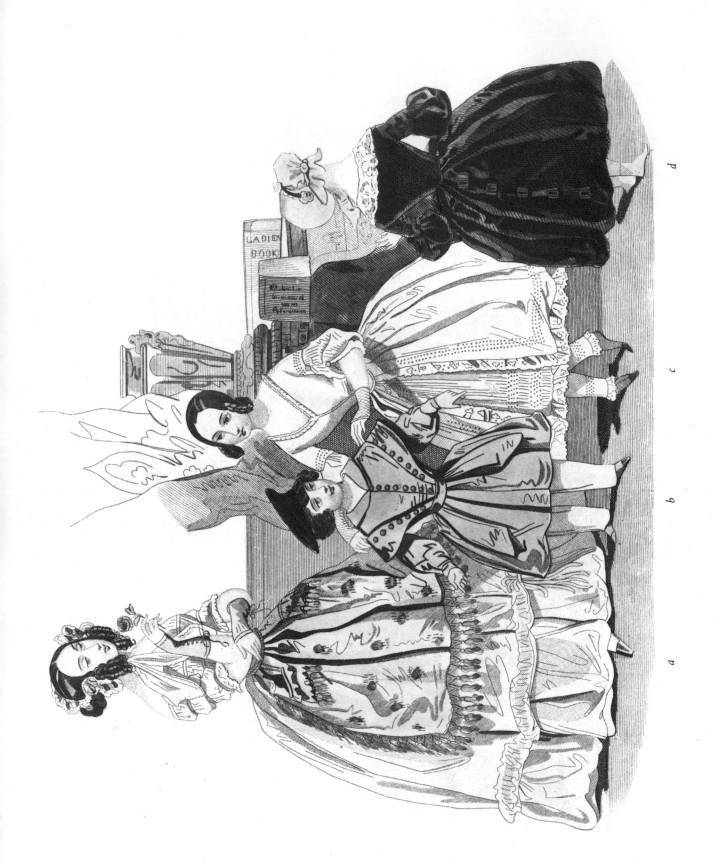

Fig. a: Dress of white silk; apron of patterned silk edged with fringe. *Fig. b:* Boy's costume of green silk; red cap. *Fig. c:* Girl's dress of white cotton open in front to show petticoat. *Fig. d:* Little girl's dress of dark silk (1/41).

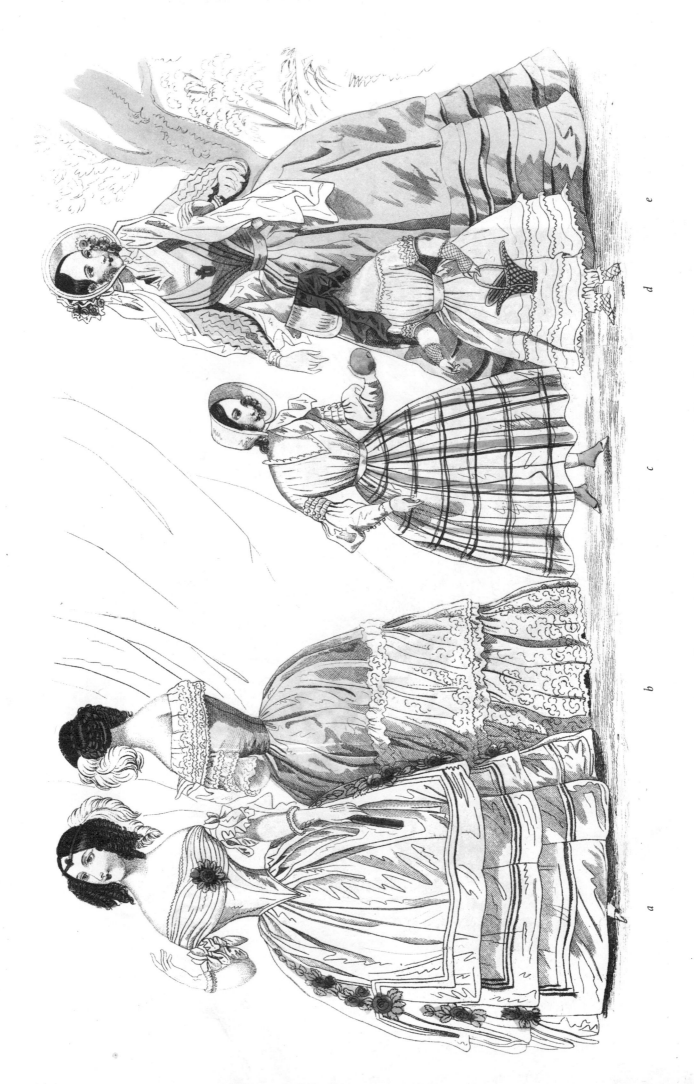

Fig. a: Evening dress of white silk trimmed with red roses. *Fig. b:* Gown of pale blue silk with lace flounces. *Fig. c:* Girl's costume; plaid skirt with white organdy blouse. *Fig. d:* Little girl's dress of white linen. *Fig. e:* Day dress of light green silk (8/41).

9

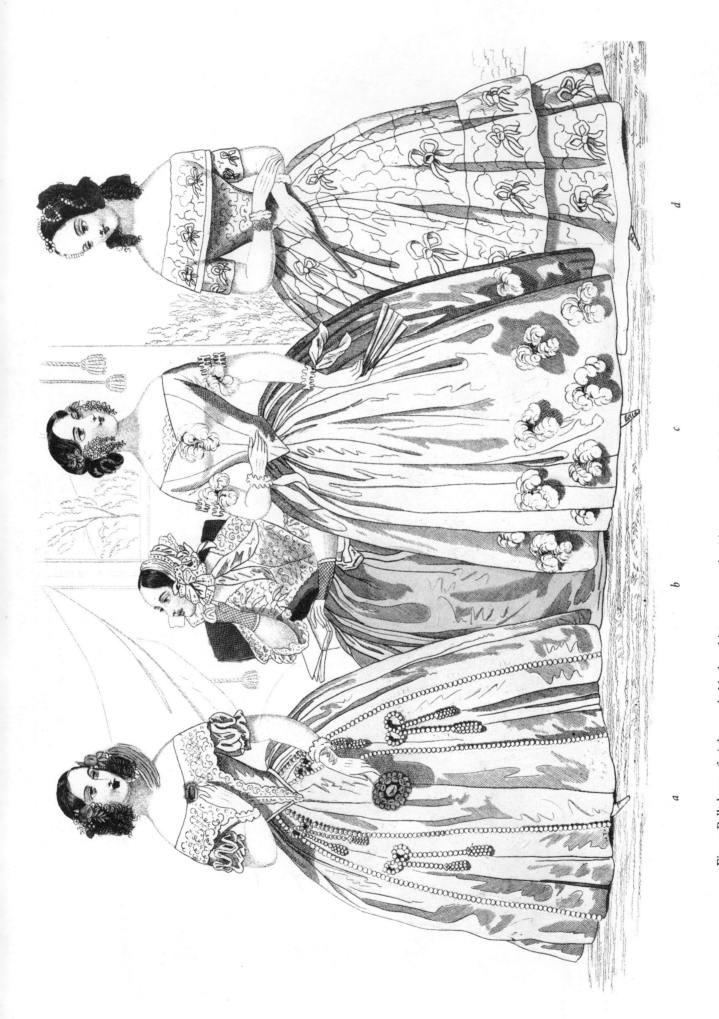

a

b

c

d

Fig. a: Ball dress of pink *gros de Naples;* skirt ornamented with pearls; white kid gloves; white satin shoes. *Fig. b:* Dress of straw-colored *poult-de-soie* shot with white, worn with lace cape. *Fig. c:* Dress of pale green satin; bodice and skirt ornamented with bou-

quets of feathers. *Fig. d:* Dress of figured gauze over white satin; skirt has two deep tucks ornamented with ribbon bows; white kid gloves with a quilling of satin ribbon at top (1/42).

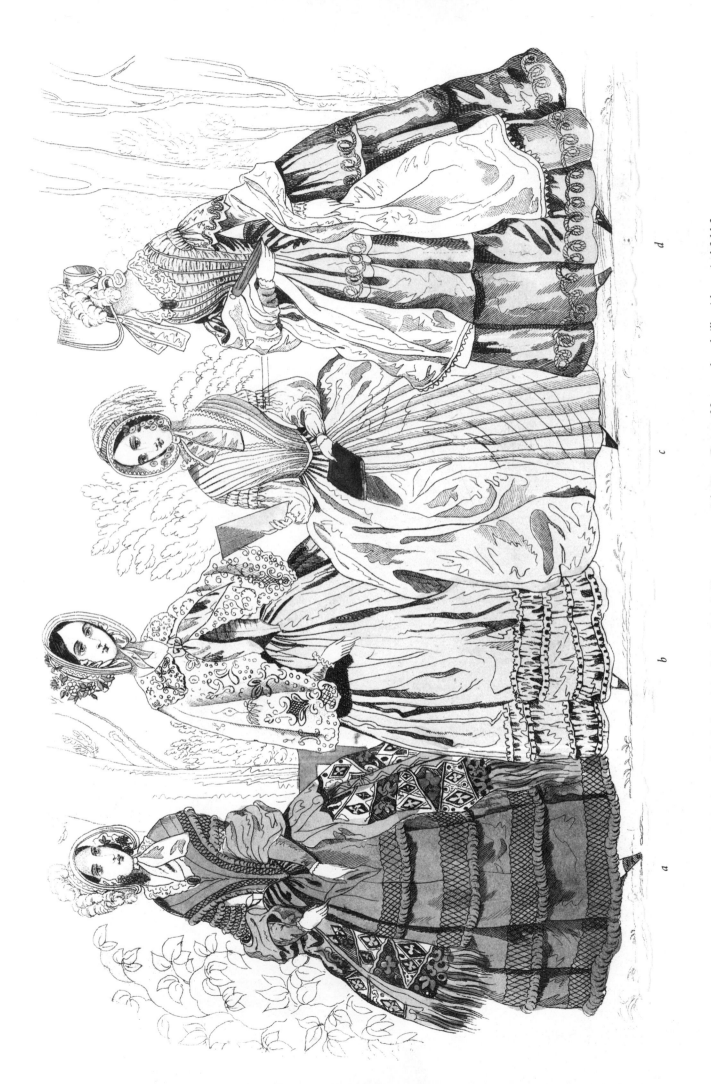

Fig. a: Promenade dress of shaded moiré, pink and dark lilac trimmed with rows of fringes; amber scarf embroidered in a Moravian pattern; bonnet of white gauze. *Fig. b*: Dress of plain colored silk; cape of figured lace lined with blue; bonnet of transparent material. *Fig. c*: Dress of fancy colored silk with vertical fold from neck to hem in front; rose-colored bonnet. *Fig. d*: Promenade dress of moiré, pink and dark lilac ornamented with scrolls of silk cord; transparent bonnet of pale primrose (10/42).

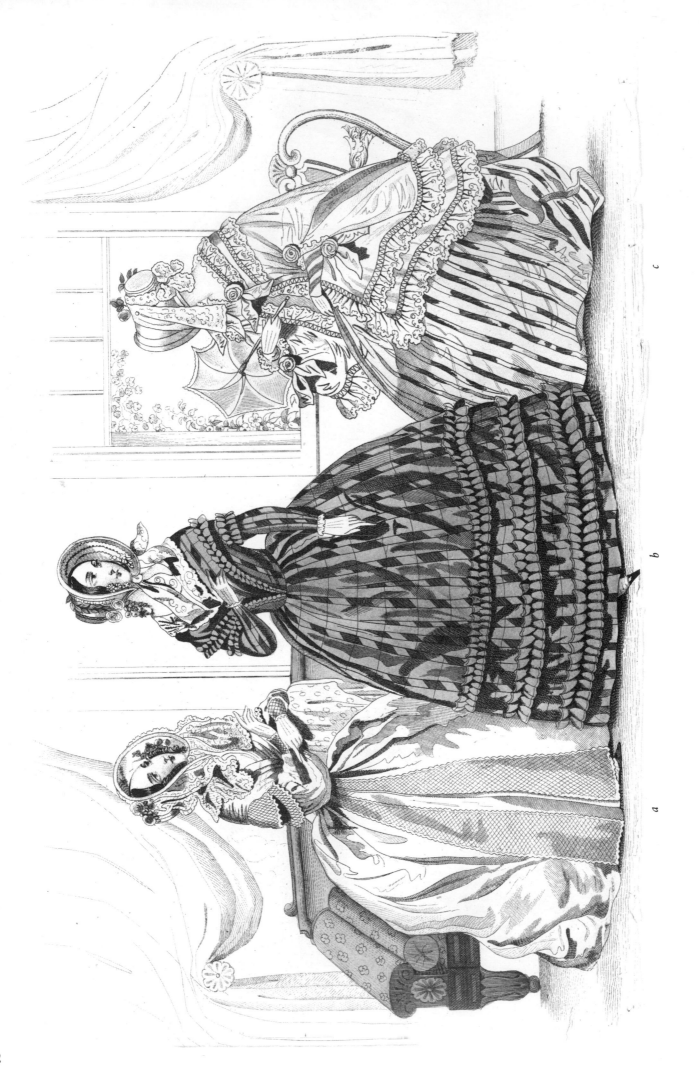

Fig a: Dress of white silk. *Fig. b:* Day dress of light brown striped and crossbarred in black. *Fig. c:* Gown of pale pink striped in black; short mantle of white trimmed with lace, pink roses, and ribbons; pale green parasol (5/43).

a

b

c

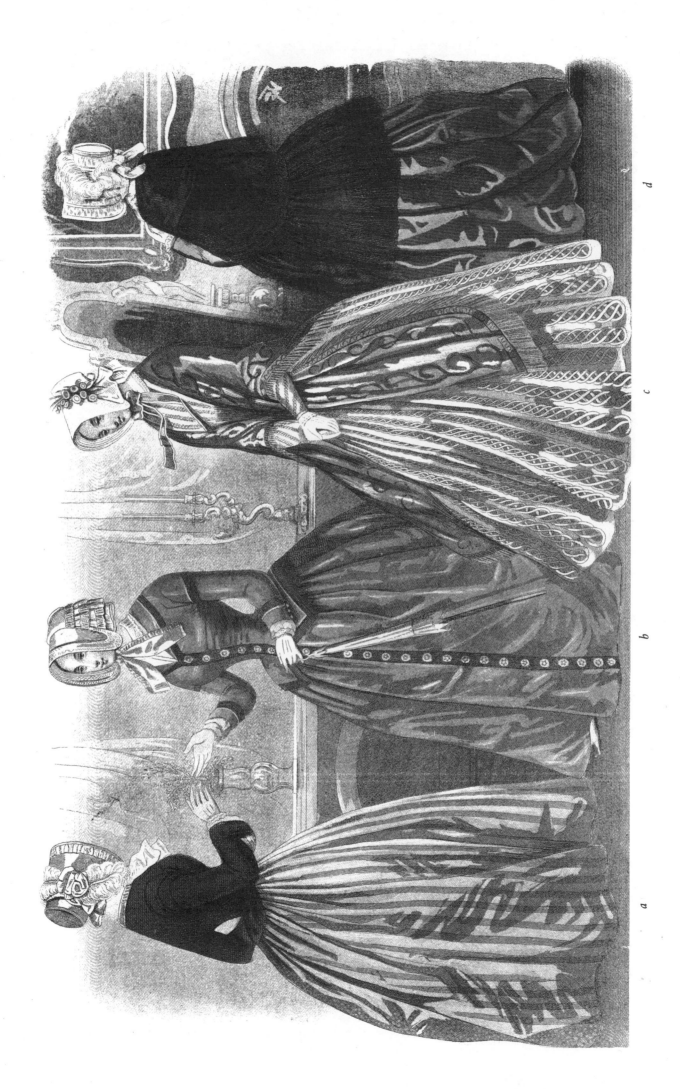

Fig. a: Skirt of striped blue-green silk with black fitted jacket. *Fig. b:* Two-piece dress of mauve silk with edging of braid; pale pink bonnet; pale blue parasol. *Fig. c:* Pink silk gown with graduated patterned stripes; green silk mantelet; pale yellow bonnet. *Fig. d:* Short cloak of black silk worn over dress of bright blue silk; white silk bonnet (10/45).

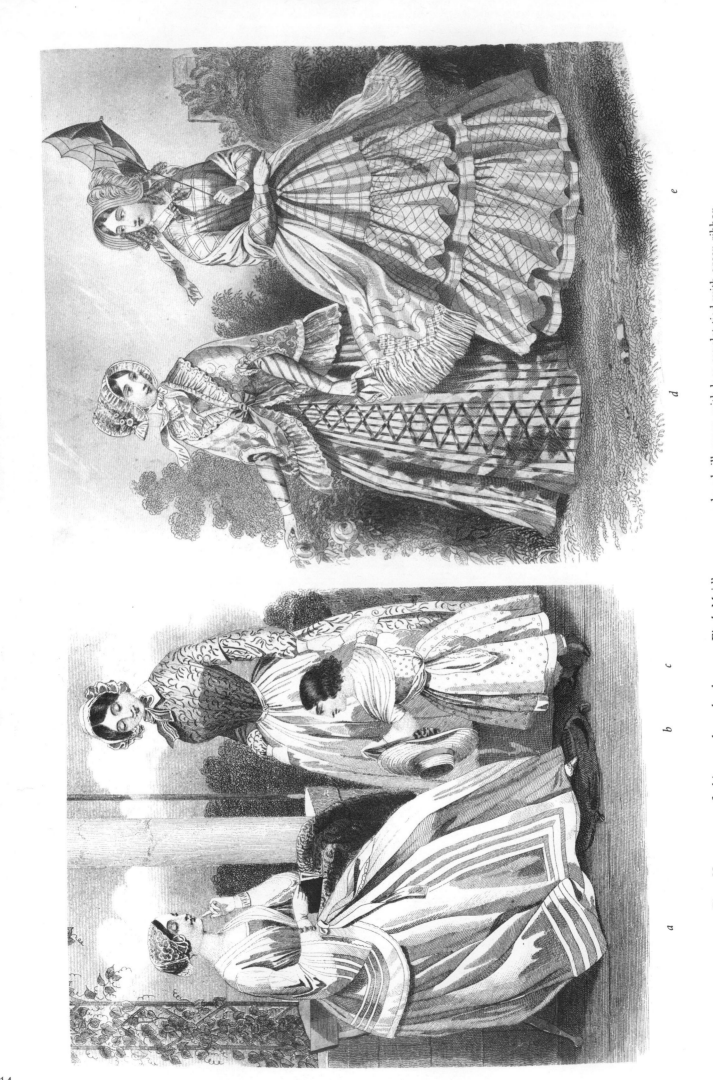

14

Fig. a: Home gown of white over lavender; lace cap. *Fig. b:* Maid's gown of patterned cotton; plain white apron. *Fig. c:* Child's gown of dotted material; wide-brimmed straw hat (5/48). *Fig. d:* Dress of rose-colored silk worn with lace capelet tied with green ribbon. *Fig. e:* Dress of slate-blue crossbarred silk; white silk fringed shawl; pink bonnet; green parasol; white gloves (6/48).

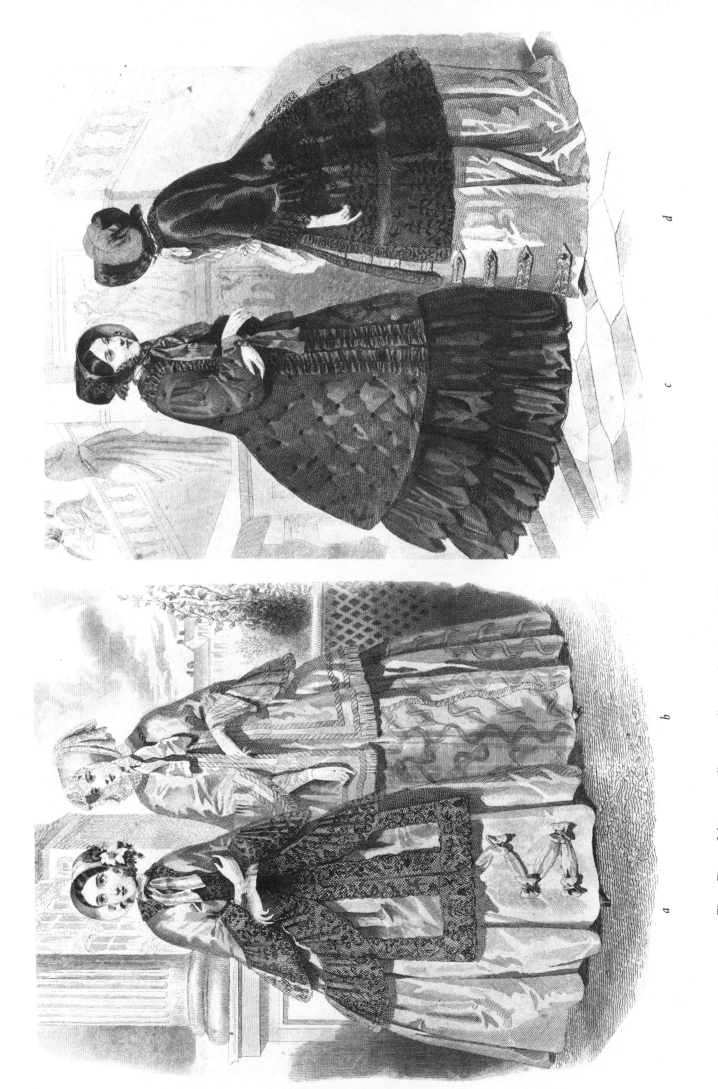

Fig. a: Dress of slate-gray silk; green silk mantelet trimmed with lace; white bonnet with pink plaid ribbons. *Fig. b:* Dress of pale pink patterned in light green; short cloak of pink taffeta; bonnet of pink silk and white lace. *Fig. c:* Black padded cloak; dress of dark green silk. *Fig. d:* Claret velvet cloak trimmed with black lace; matching bonnet; slate-gray gown (1848).

15

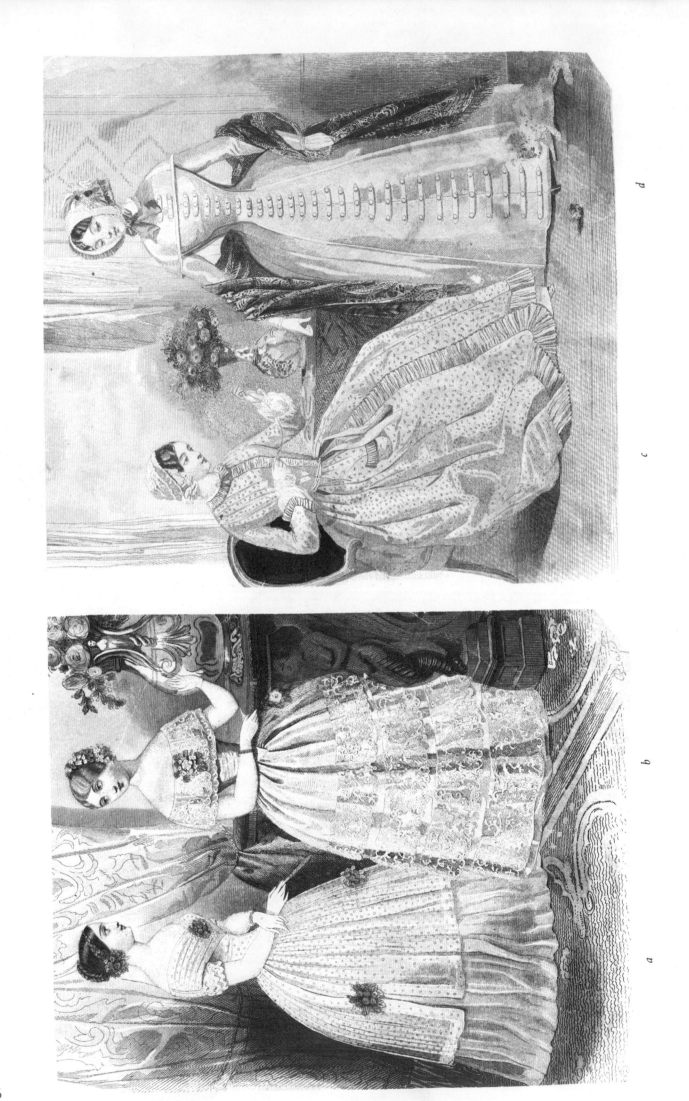

16

Fig. a: Evening gown of white dotted fabric trimmed with bouquets of small roses. *Fig. b*: Evening gown of white silk with white lace flounce (2/49). *Fig. c*: House gown of dotted pink cloth. *Fig. d*: Shaped one-piece gown of white fabric worn with cashmere shawl; white silk bonnet with blue ribbons (3/49).

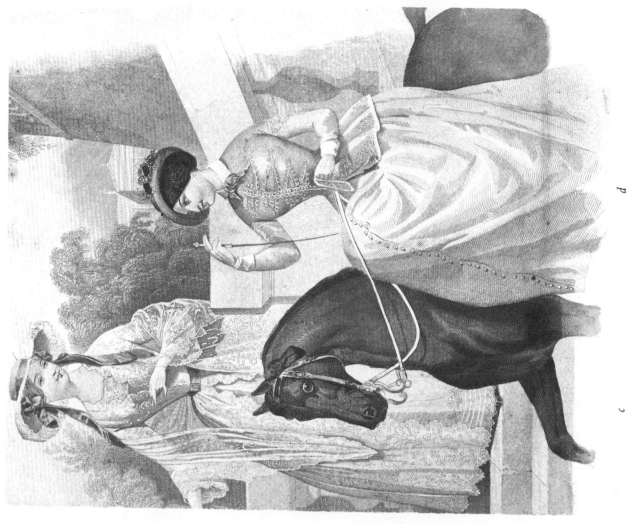

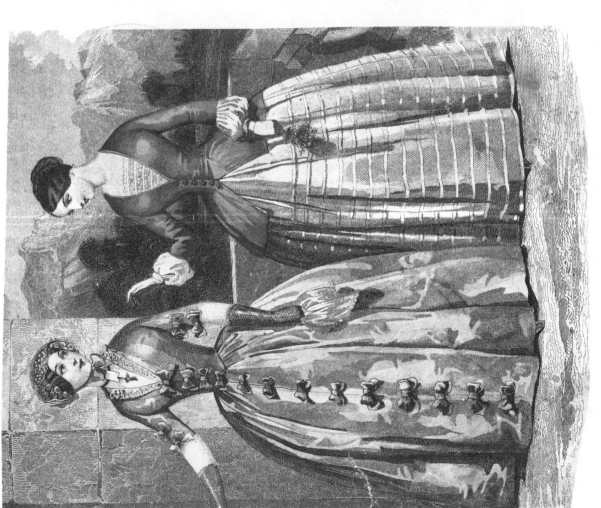

Fig. a: Short-sleeved gown of rose changeable silk; lace cap with rose ribbons and flowers; black net mittens. *Fig. b:* Green silk basque worn with pale gray silk (4/49). *Fig. c:* Summer dress of white cotton open in front to show petticoat; green silk belt; broad-brimmed hat with green ribbons. *Fig. d:* Equestrian costume, light tan skirt and buff-colored bodice trimmed with braid; blue lining and bow tie; straw hat (1849).

17

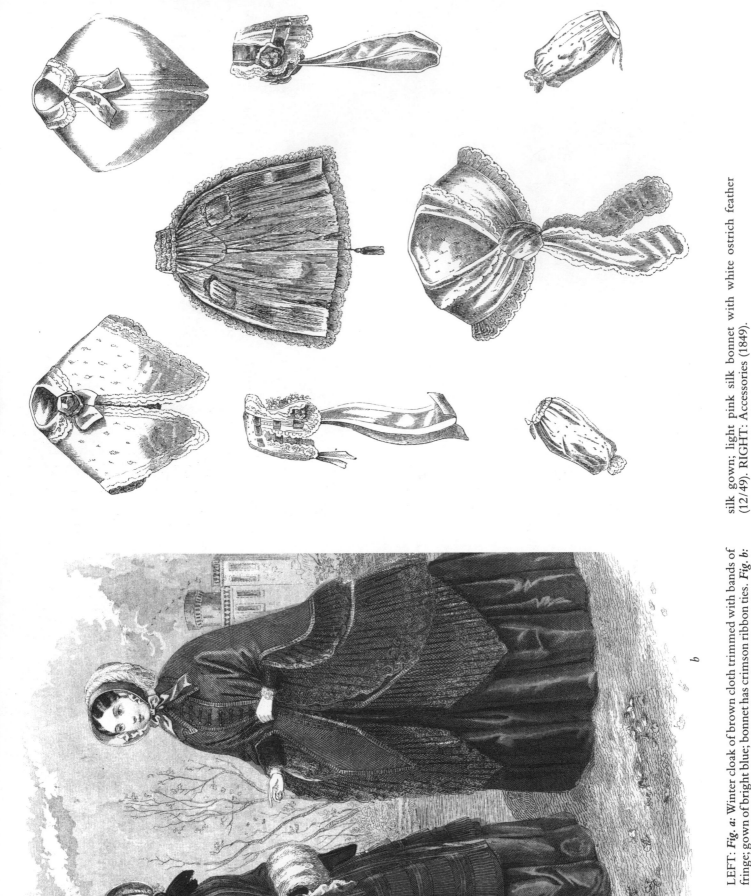

18

LEFT: *Fig. a:* Winter cloak of brown cloth trimmed with bands of fringe; gown of bright blue; bonnet has crimson ribbon ties. *Fig. b:* Dark green cloak edged with black lace; claret-colored changeable silk gown; light pink silk bonnet with white ostrich feather (12/49). RIGHT: Accessories (1849).

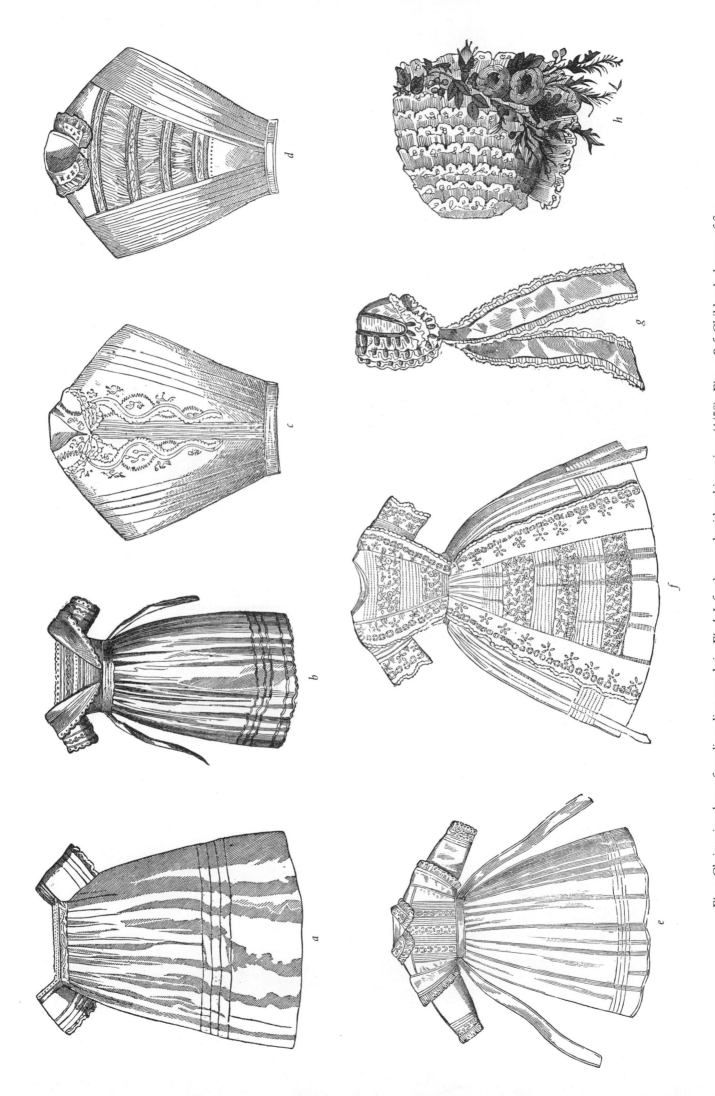

Fig. a: Christening dress of muslin or linen cambric. *Fig. b:* Infant's robe with waist *en chemisette* with edgings and insertion of embroidered cambric (2/50). *Fig. c:* Chemisette of embroidered muslin. *Fig. d:* Chemisette with puffs of fine Swiss muslin between embroidered insertions (4/50). *Figs. e & f:* Children's dresses of fine cambric (7/50). *Fig. g:* Breakfast cap of muslin with embroidered frills. *Fig. h:* Cap for a dinner dress or evening parties made of rows of lace and trimmed with flowers (5/50).

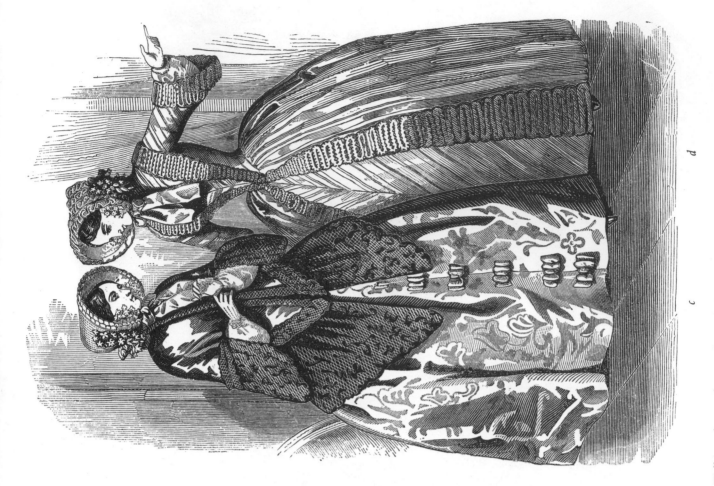

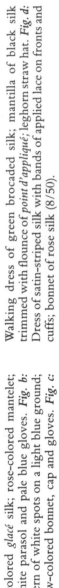

c
d

Walking dress of green brocaded silk; mantilla of black silk trimmed with flounce of *point d'appliqué*; leghorn straw hat. *Fig. d:* Dress of satin-striped silk with bands of applied lace on fronts and cuffs; bonnet of rose silk (8/50).

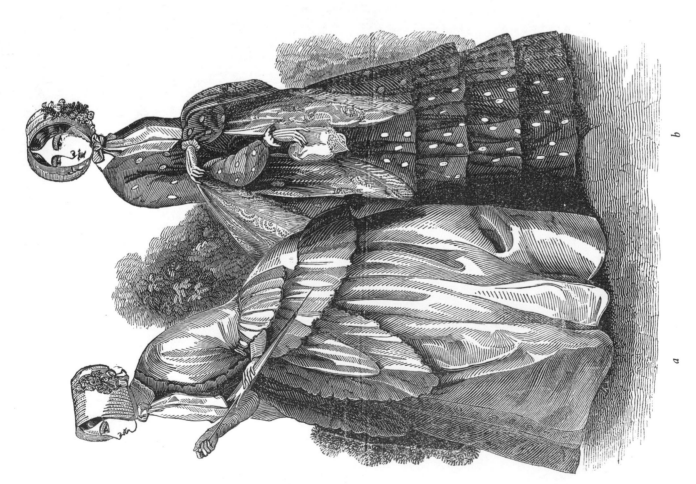

a
b

Fig. a: Dress of slate-colored *glacé* silk; rose-colored mantelet; French chip bonnet; white parasol and pale blue gloves. *Fig. b:* Robe of *barège* in a pattern of white spots on a light blue ground; white crape shawl; straw-colored bonnet, cap and gloves. *Fig. c:*

20

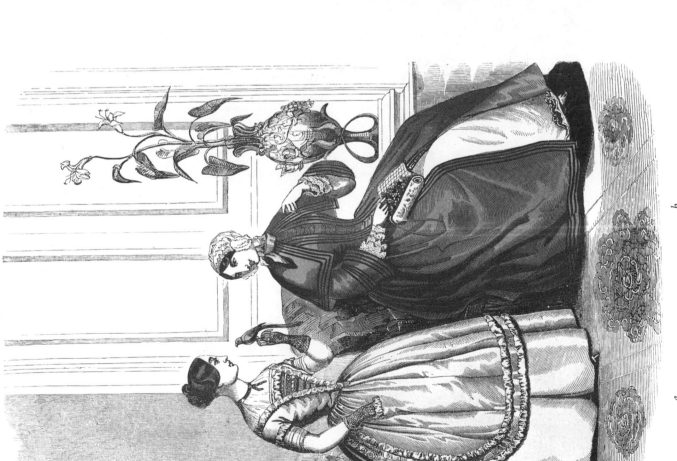

Honiton lace; chemisette of rich needlework; veil of Honiton lace fastened with white roses. *Fig. d:* Bridal dress of white brocaded silk; chemisette of lighter silk; wreath of orange buds and white roses confines a simple tulle veil (8/5c).

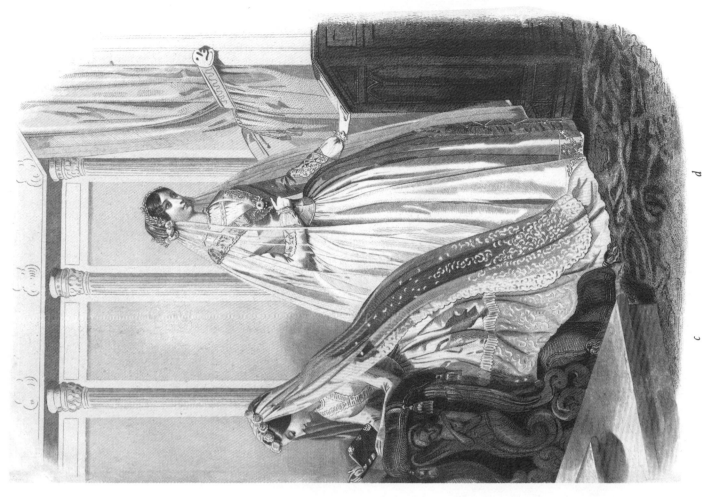

Fig. a: Home dress for a young lady of dove-colored silk; apron of green silk; chemisette of plain lace. *Fig. b:* Robe of white cambric and wrapper of garnet-colored silk or cashmere; worn with break-fast cap (8/50). *Fig. c:* Bridal robe of white satin with a flounce of

21

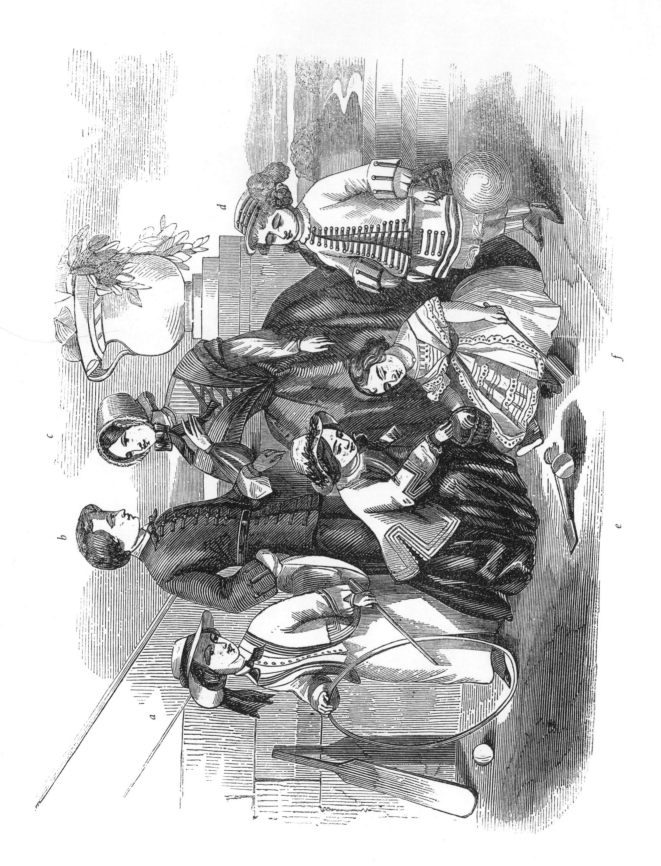

Fig. a: Young boy's suit of cloth trimmed with braid; leghorn straw hat. *Fig. b:* Boy's suit of cloth trimmed with braid and silk buttons. *Fig. c:* Schoolgirl's dress of cashmere *de baize*; chemisette of fine muslin; cottage straw bonnet. *Fig. d:* Little boy's skirt and jacket of cloth trimmed with contrasting braid; white muslin pantalettes. *Fig. e:* Little girl's dress of plain dark cashmere with a sacque of blue *mousseline de laine*; chip hat. *Fig. f:* Baby sister's dress of white muslin (9/50).

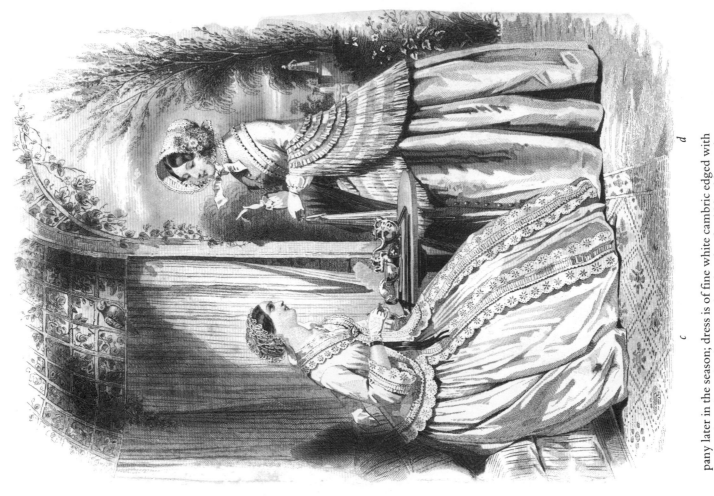

d

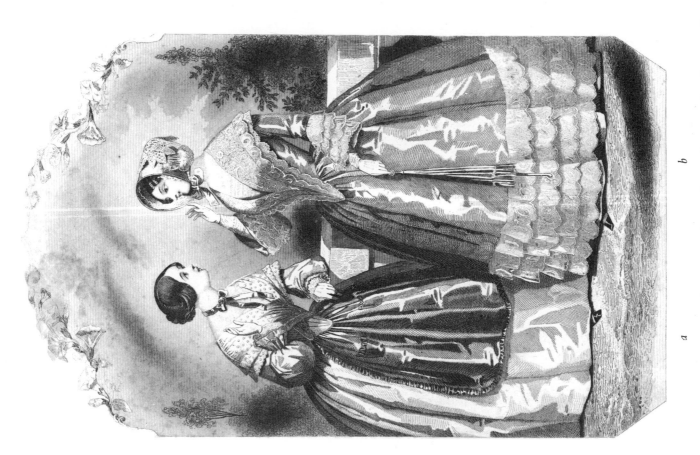

a

b

c

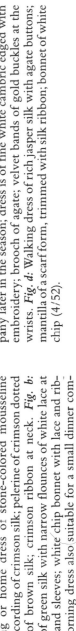

Fig. a: Morning or home dress of stone-colored mousseline
trimmed with a cording of crimson silk; pelerine of crimson dotted
muslin; apron of brown silk; crimson ribbon at neck. Fig. b:
Carriage dress of green silk with narrow flounces of white lace at
hem on bodice and sleeves; white chip bonnet with lace and ribbons. Fig. c: Morning dress also suitable for a small dinner company later in the season; dress is of fine white cambric edged with
embroidery; brooch of agate; velvet bands of gold buckles at the
wrists. Fig. d: Walking dress of rich jasper silk with agate buttons;
mantilla of a scarf form, trimmed with silk ribbon; bonnet of white
chip (4/52).

23

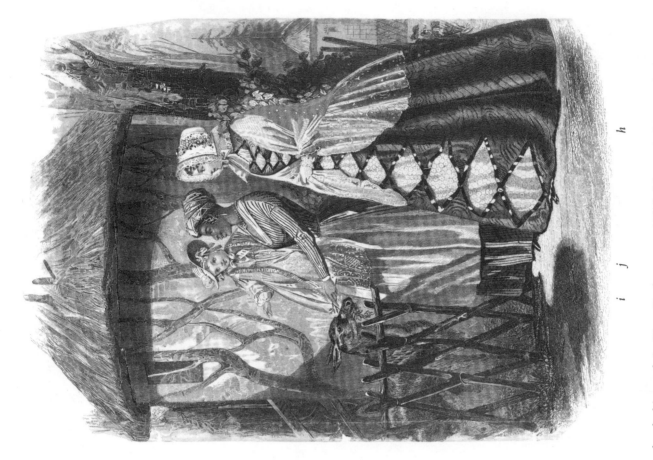

i   j   h

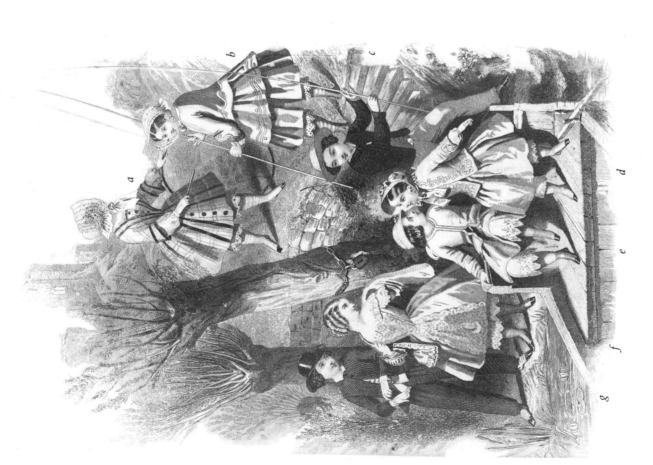

g   f   e   d

Fig. a: Child's walking dress of pink cashmere with light black satin bar and edged with black velvet ribbon. *Fig. b*: Dress of pale violet India silk; small cloak of gray merino with blue embroidery; pink bonnet; gray gaiters. *Fig. c*: Boy's suit with gray trousers; dark green jacket. *Fig. d*: Girl's dress of pale blue mousseline or cashmere; sacque of white merino. *Fig. e*: Boy's dress; buff sacque and skirt; white linen trousers with embroidered edge; bronze gaiters with patent-leather tips. *Fig. f*: Dress and pantalettes of embroi-

dered white cambric. *Fig. g*: Boy's costume with dark brown jacket and trousers; white vest; beaver hat; blue-and-white stockings; patent-leather slippers (5/52). *Fig. h*: Walking dress of dark *moire d'antique*, a very rich silk with diamond-shaped cutouts; light mantle of India muslin; white silk bonnet. *Fig. i*: Child's dress of embroidered cambric; leghorn straw hat; mantle of pink cashmere. *Fig. j*: Nurse has a brown stuff dress; white apron and brilliant madras neckerchief twisted about her head (10/52).

24

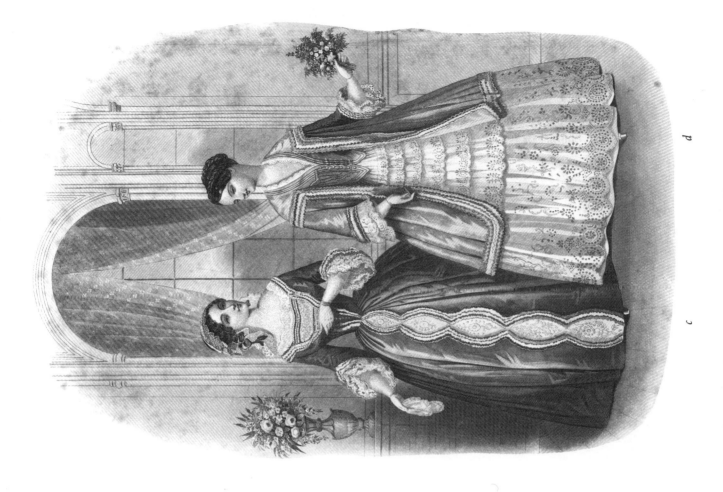

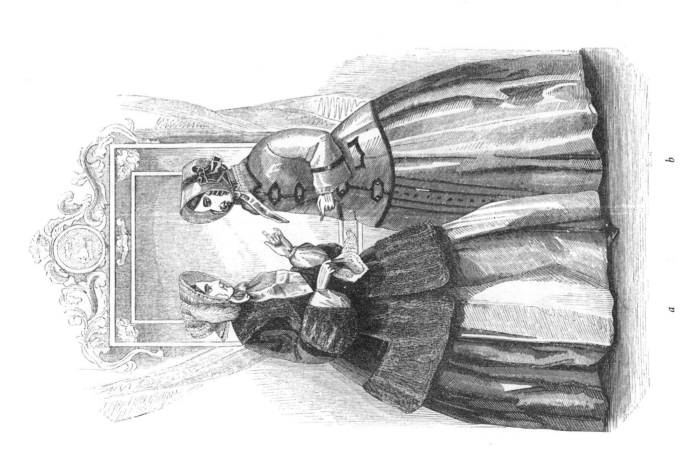

Fig. a: Sacque mantle of dark green velvet, padded and trimmed with stone marten. Dress of stone-colored *moire d'antique. Fig. b:* Traveling dress; pelisse and sacque of mole-colored habit cloth; trimmed with velvet bands; matching velvet bonnet (11/52). *Fig. c* Evening dress of pale violet silk; trimmings are narrow puffs of ribbon; double fall of lace serves as undersleeves; headdress of lace and pink ribbons. *Fig. d:* Dinner dress of cambric with embroidered flounces; vest, or gilet corsage, of green watered silk; opera cloak of straw-colored cashmere (12/52).

25

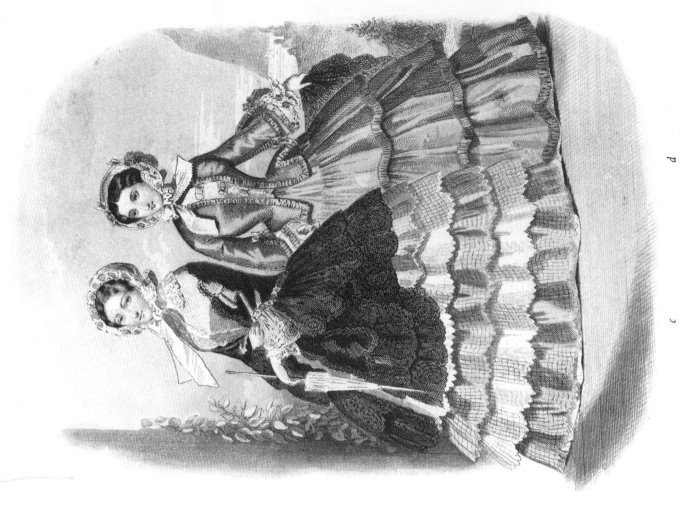

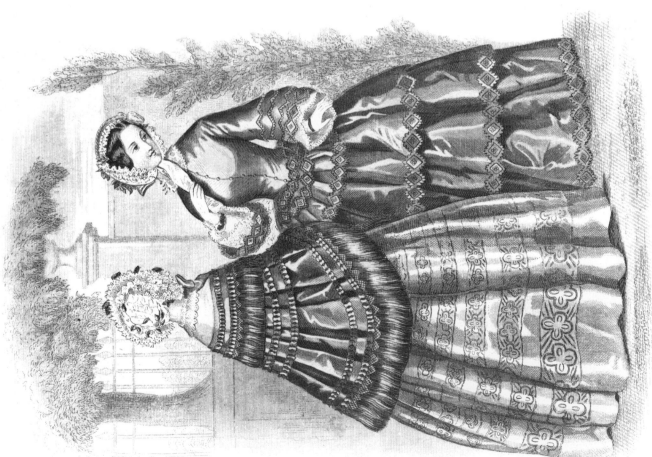

Fig. a: Carriage dress of silver-gray *poult-de-soie;* skirt trimmed with rows of galoon and raised black velvet figures on satin ground; mantle of green silk; white silk bonnet. *Fig. b:* Walking dress of violet-colored mousseline or cashmere; leghorn hat; inside cap of blonde lace (3/55). *Fig. c:* Walking dress of two shades of

organdy; pink belt ribbon and small pearl buckle; Spanish mantilla; white silk bonnet; cap of blonde lace. *Fig. d:* Walking dress of stone-colored taffeta; skirt with three deep flounces edged with a quilling of green satin ribbon; English straw bonnet; bonnet cap of blonde lace and pink ribbon (4/55).

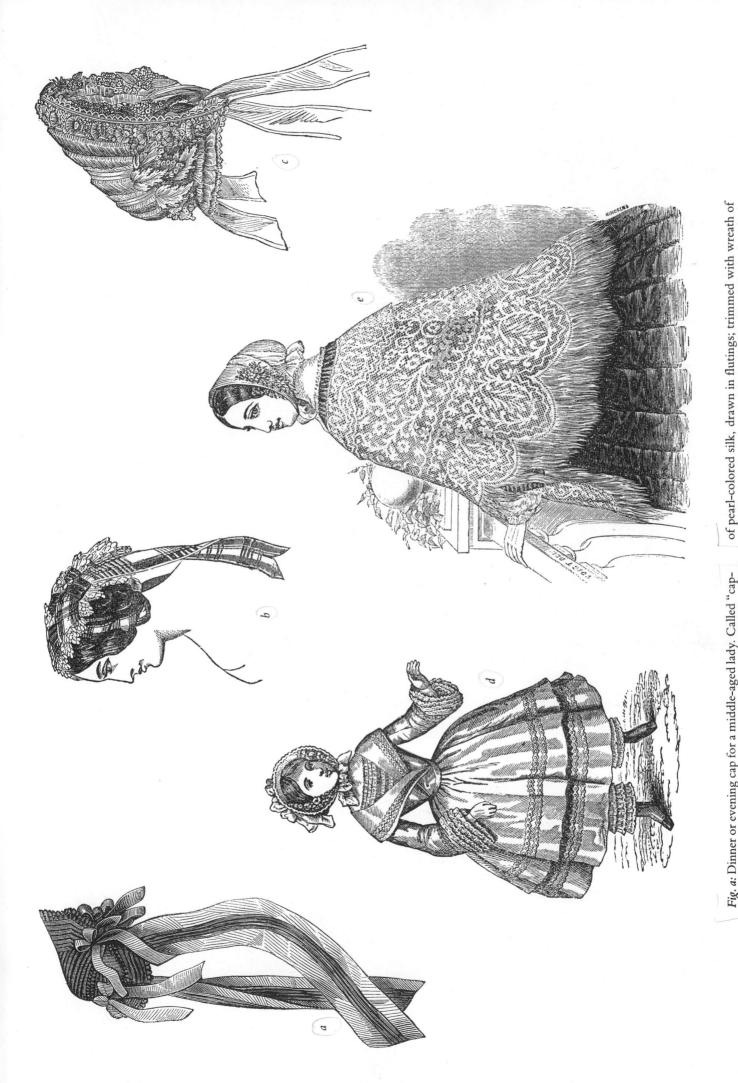

Fig. a: Dinner or evening cap for a middle-aged lady. Called "cap-bonnet," it is made of rows of black velvet ribbon on net. It could also be made in white (6/55). *Fig. b:* Intended for a young girlish face, this cap is of Maltese lace with bands of black velvet ribbons; trimming is *ruban écossais* and black velvet (11/54). *Fig. c:* Dress cap of pearl-colored silk, drawn in flutings; trimmed with wreath of velvet leaves, flowers and ribbons (6/55). *Fig. d:* Dress for a little girl under the age of twelve, of pink *barège* trimmed with silk braid; pantalettes with crimped frills, lace or muslin (8/55). *Fig. e:* Mantilla, an appliqué of white taffeta on white lace (8/54).

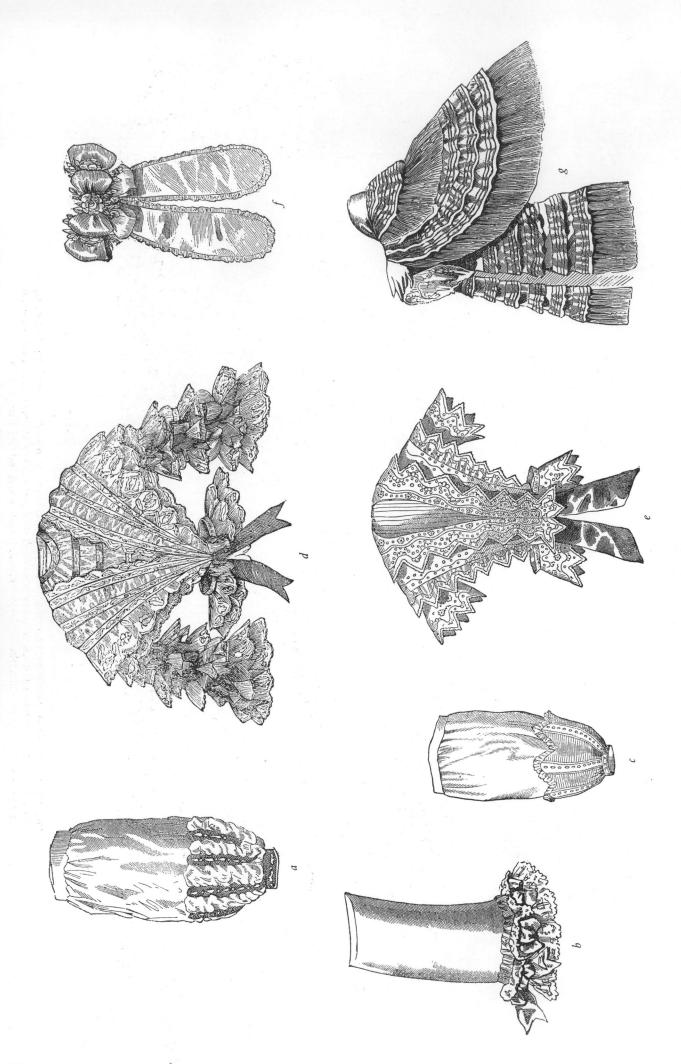

Fig. a: Spring undersleeve of muslin with rows of lace and ribbon bows. *Fig. b:* Summer undersleeve with lower puffs separated by bands of lace (6/55). *Fig. c:* Sleeve of delicate imported muslin; with plainer insertion, it could be worn for mourning (9/54). *Fig. d:* Jacket intended for full dress of dotted Swiss muslin (10/54).

Fig. e: Basque of rich lace to be worn with low-necked evening dress. *Fig. f:* "Court bows" for sash (11/54). *Fig. g:* "Omer" mantle of ruffles bordered with velvet satin ribbon or braid and a heavy fringe. This mantle can be made of silk or thin material such as *barège* or tissue, etc. (6/55).

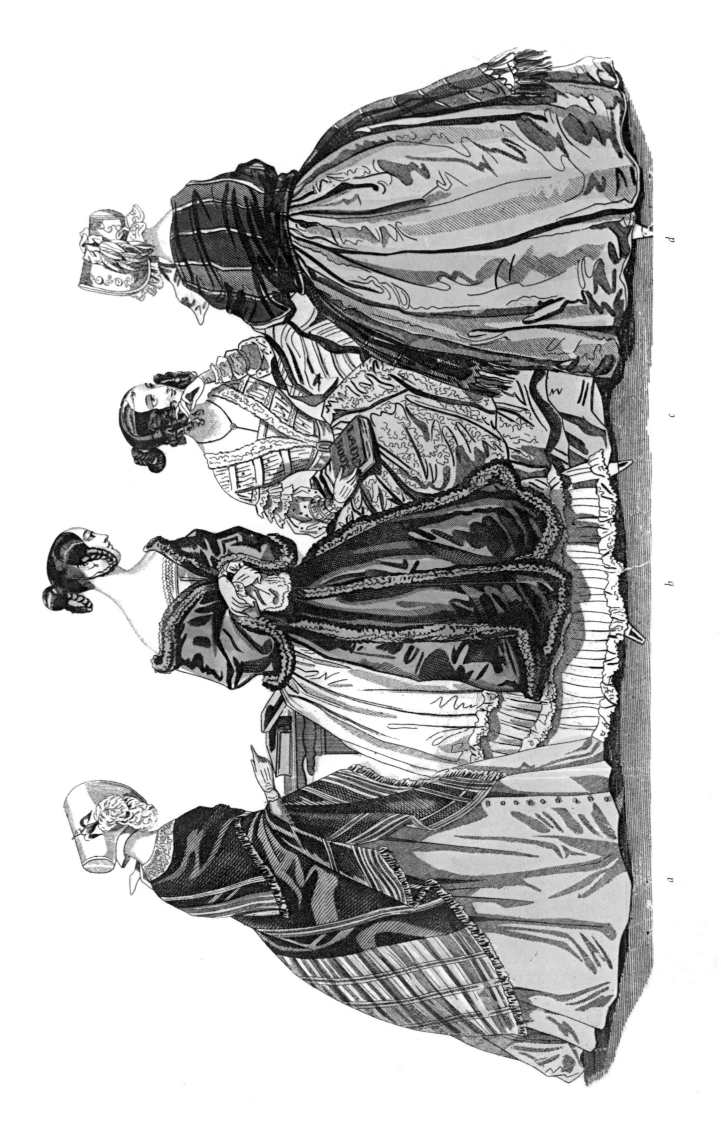

Fig. a: Dress with front opening of fawn-colored silk worn with large square shawl of wool. *Fig. b:* Evening gown of white silk; mantelet of black taffeta. *Fig. c:* Skirt of green silk worn with chemisette of white organdy. *Fig. d:* Dress of changeable silk; shawl of red, brown, green and white stripes (2/41).

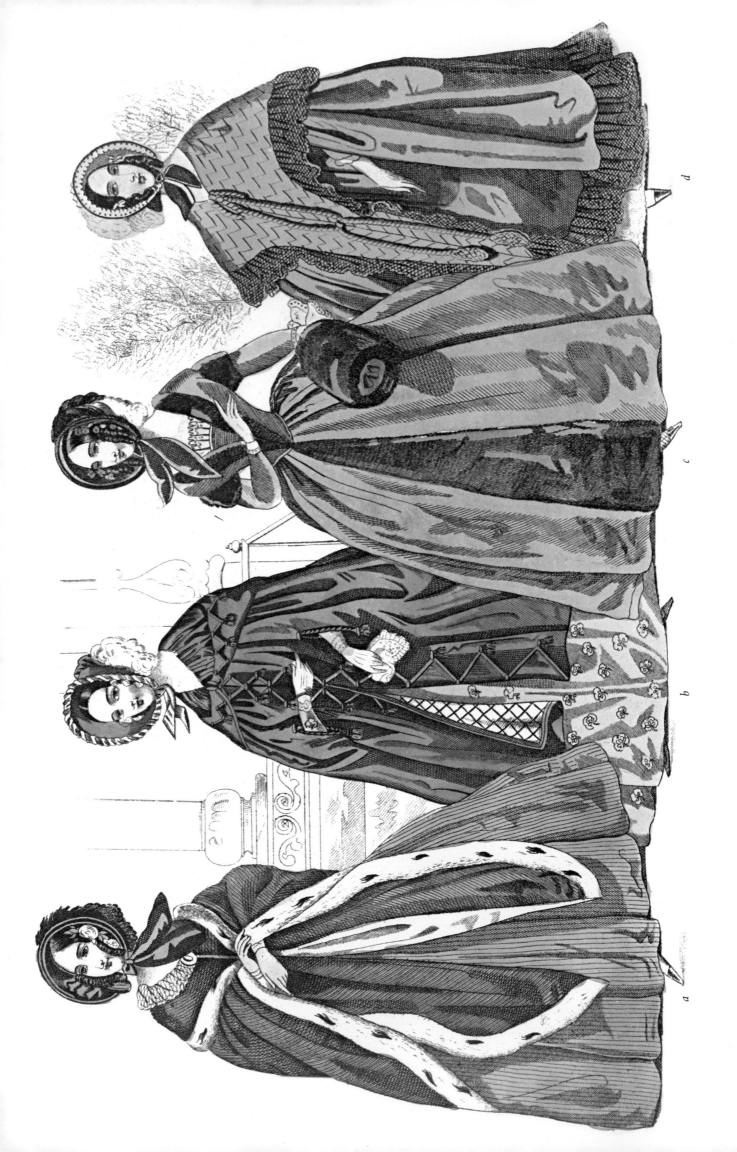

Fig. a: Dress of striped plain silk; large velvet shawl trimmed with ermine; bonnet of dark velvet. *Fig. b:* Dress of rich silk; mantle of velvet lined with plaid silk. *Fig. c:* Walking dress of silk trimmed with sable. *Fig. d:* Full-length satin cloak trimmed with rich lace and silk cord; satin bonnet (12/41).

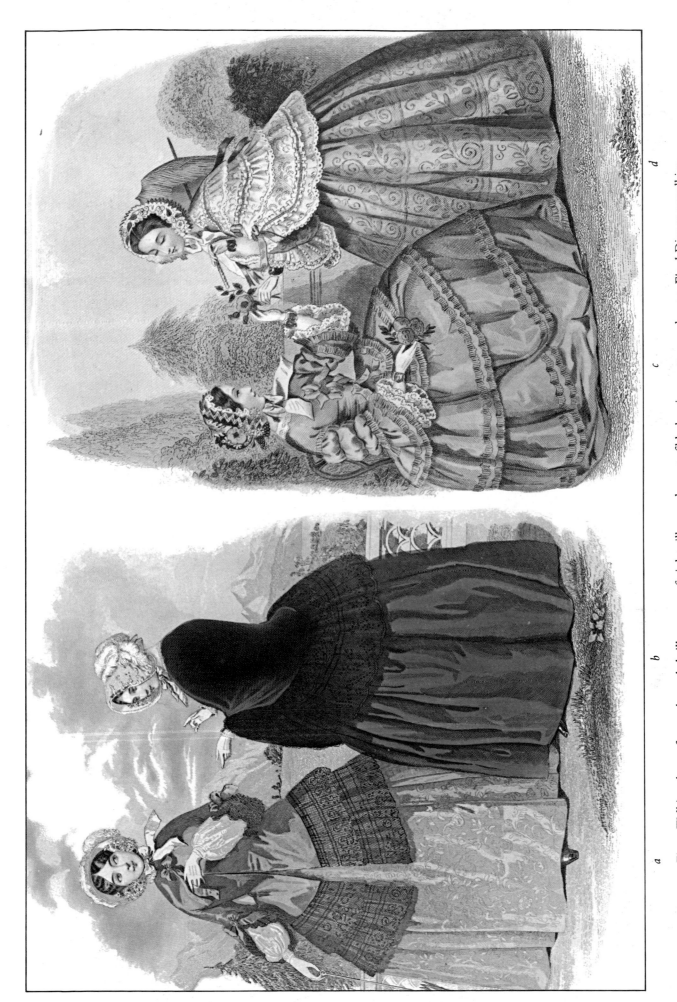

Fig. a: Walking dress of green brocaded silk; sacque of violet silk and black lace; bonnet of white. *Fig. b:* Dress of garnet velvet; mantilla of matching garnet and black lace; blue silk bonnet (10/50). *Fig. c:* Walking dress of fawn-colored silk; jacket corsage fastened by knots of satin ribbon; collar and cuffs of Maltese lace;

bonnet of black guipure, straw and crape. *Fig. d:* Dinner or walking dress of patterned blue organdy; small scarf mantelet of embroidered lace or muslin; bonnet of fancy straw, blonde lace and crape flowers (6/55).

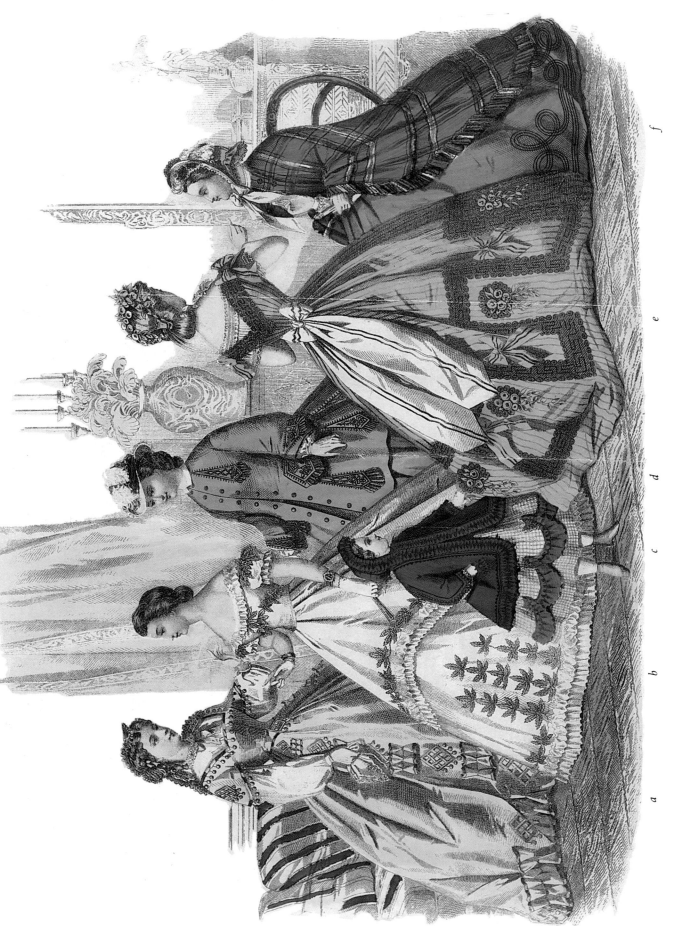

Fig. a: Dinner dress of pearl-gray silk trimmed with ornaments of gold-colored chenille cord and chenille drop buttons. *Fig. b:* Evening dress of heavy white corded silk trimmed with black lace leaves. *Fig. c:* Child's costume. Red Riding Hood sack of scarlet flannel; dress of checked silk trimmed with Imperial blue silk. *Fig. d:* Walking dress of smoke-gray poplin; trimmings of rich passementerie; white chip hat with scarlet velvet and white plumes. *Fig. e:* Gown of lilac silk with a fancy lace design on skirt; sash of white silk trimmed with black velvet. *Fig. f:* Walking dress of brown alpaca with black-braid trim; fancy plaid wrap with chenille fringe (4/64).

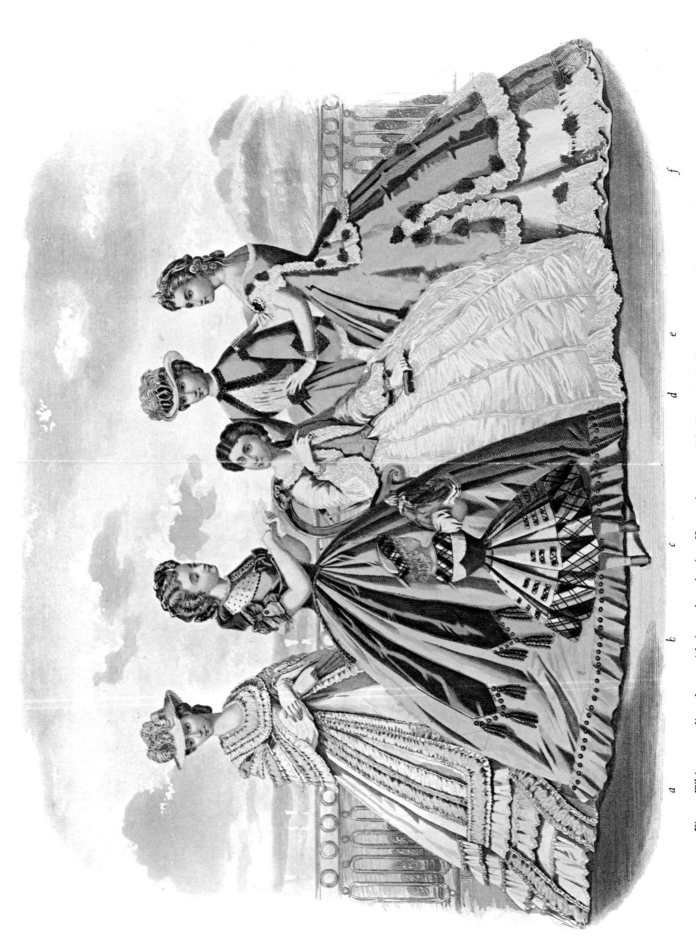

Fig. a: White grenadine dress with lavender-edged ruffles and puffs; narrow matching mantle; hat of rice straw with violet and white plumes. *Fig. b:* Dress of buff silk with black silk and large chenille tassels and drop buttons; coiffure has loops of scarlet and black ribbon. *Fig. c:* Child's dress of oyster-white alpaca trimmed with brilliant plaid silk. *Fig. d:* Dress of French muslin with a bright blue vest. *Fig. e:* Dress of pink percale printed in a design to resemble lace. *Fig. f:* Ball dress; underdress of white *glacé* silk; overdress of green silk trimmed with point lace and black thread lace leaves (7/64).

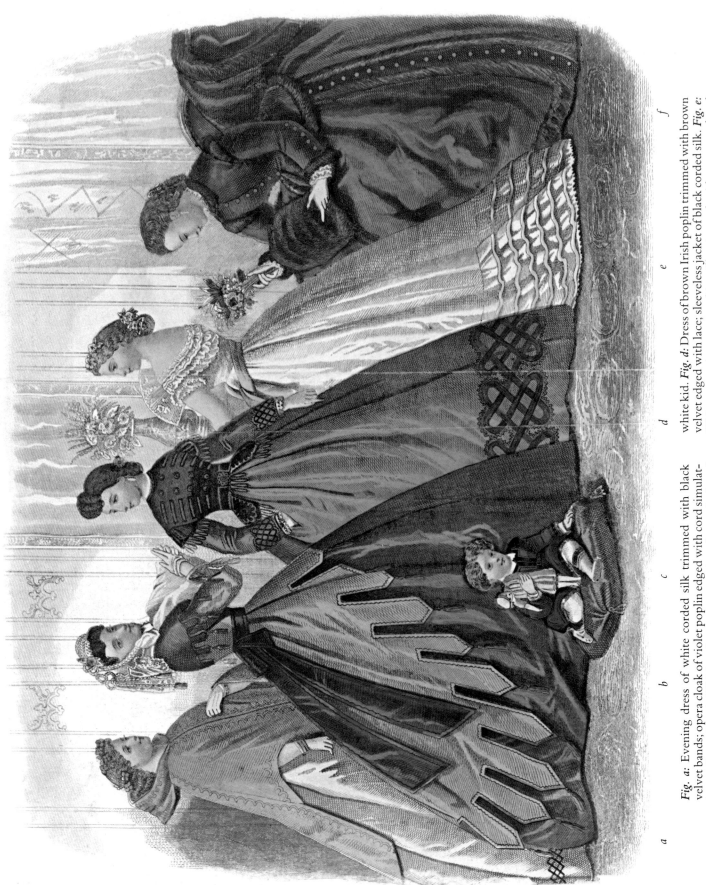

Fig. a: Evening dress of white corded silk trimmed with black velvet bands; opera cloak of violet poplin edged with cord simulating scallops. *Fig. b:* Visiting dress of *gros grains* of two shades of blue; bonnet of white satin and gold chenille. *Fig. c:* Little boy's suit of crimson poplin trimmed with brown velvet; Polish boots of white kid. *Fig. d:* Dress of brown Irish poplin trimmed with brown velvet edged with lace; sleeveless jacket of black corded silk. *Fig. e:* White crape dress over white silk trimmed with canary-colored silk. *Fig. f:* Promenade suit of purple poplin trimmed with Hudson Bay sable (12/65).

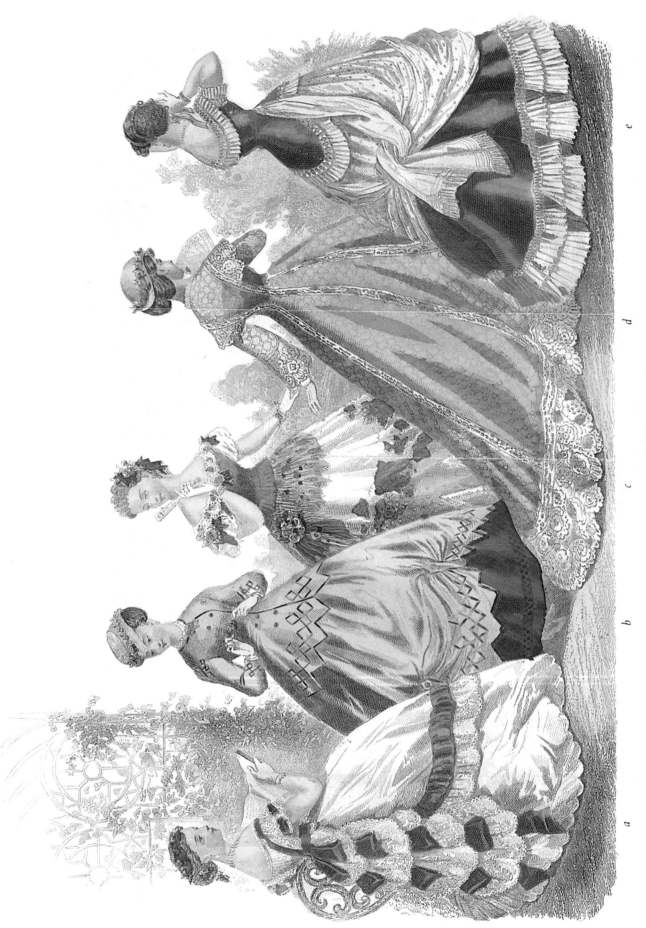

Fig. a: Costume for watering place; dress of white muslin trimmed with a flounce of embroidered muslin and a band of blue ribbon arranged to simulate overskirt; blue ribbons and lace at back. *Fig. b*: Costume for seaside; petticoat of scarlet skirting trimmed with row of black-and-white velvet; mohair dress bound in black velvet; hat of gray straw, trimmed with wreath of bright flowers. *Fig. c*: Fancy costume representing four seasons; upper part, spring shown by flowers; summer shown by grain hanging from waist; autumn by garland of grape leaves and bunches of grapes; winter by a skirt of white satin trimmed with swansdown and crystal drops. *Fig. d*: Underskirt of rose-colored silk over which is worn a dress of white gauze with rose-colored dots ornamented with Cluny lace. *Fig. e*: Dress for watering place; underskirt of blue silk; overskirt of white dotted gauze; corsage of blue silk trimmed with white silk (8/67).

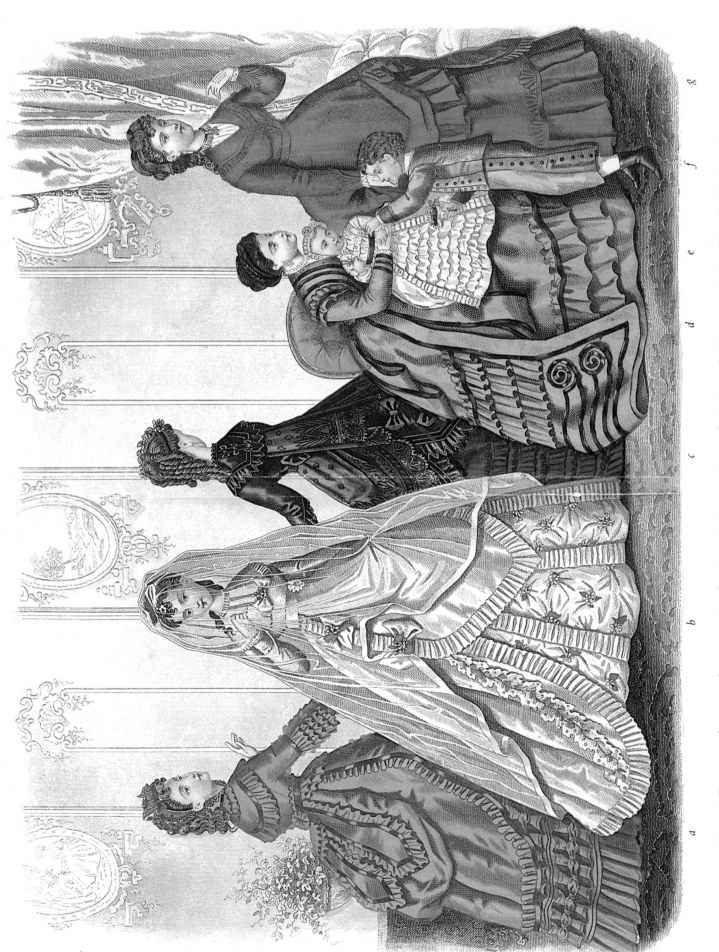

Fig. a: Walking suit of green poplin; green satin trimming. *Fig. b:* Bride's dress of corded silk; tulle-ruche trim and bouquets of flowers. *Fig. c:* Dress of blue silk with silk and lace Watteau casaque. *Fig. d:* Dress of golden-brown serge with satin trim.

Fig. e: Infant's dress of white nainsook. *Fig. f:* Suit for little boy, of gray cashmere trimmed with brown velvet; bronze kid boots. *Fig. g:* Suit of purple cloth (11/69).

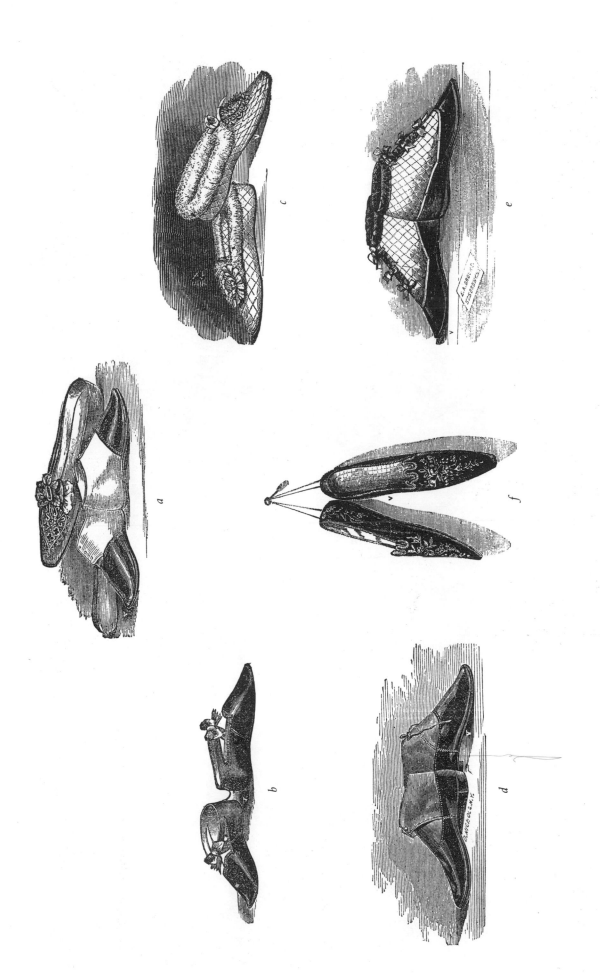

Figs. a & b: Children's shoes of patent leather, bronze morocco and glazed calfskin (8/54). *Fig. c:* Boudoir slippers of silk and satin trimmed with swansdown. *Fig. d:* Shoes for boys with rich bronze tops and patent-leather vamps (11/54). *Fig. e:* Quilted boots for girls. *Fig. f:* Boudoir or dress slippers of rich colors of velvet and chenille (2/55).

29

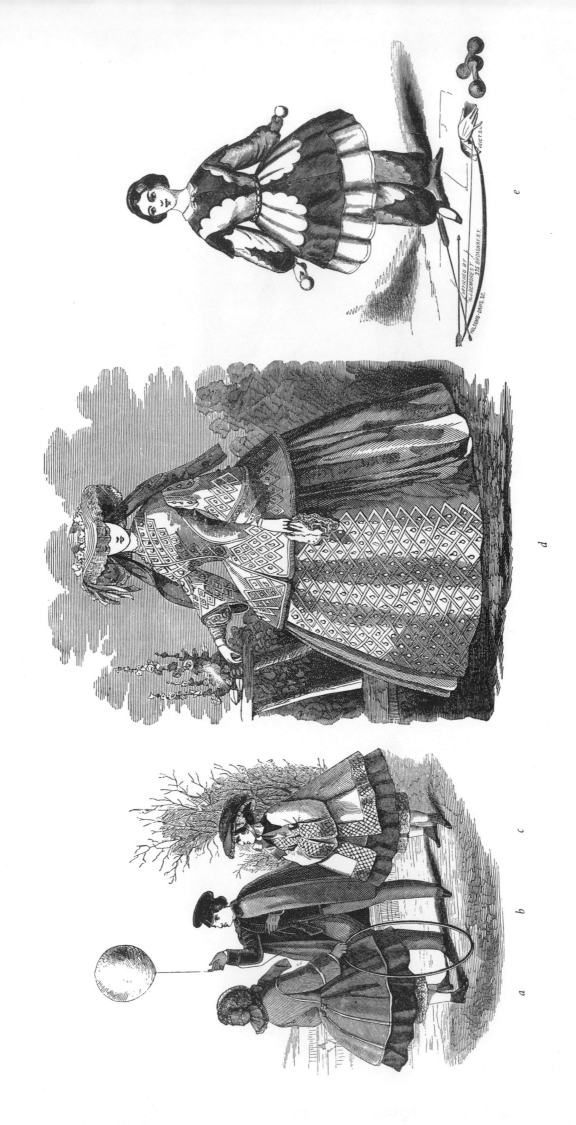

Fig. a: Little girl's costume with black silk jacket; full skirt of crimson merino; green drawn bonnet. *Fig. b:* Boy's suit of black kersey worn with cloak of brown cloth with velvet collar; flat cap of black cloth with velvet band. *Fig. c:* Street sacque of fawn-colored merino with a silk piqué border; blue cashmere dress; fawn-colored beaver hat with blonde fall and a plume (1/58). *Fig. d:* Dress for the country or watering places of white piqué trimmed with braid; Pamela straw hat with black lace demiveil (5/58). *Fig. e:* Gymnastic costume; material may be either fine flannel or French merino of any two contrasting colors (1/58).

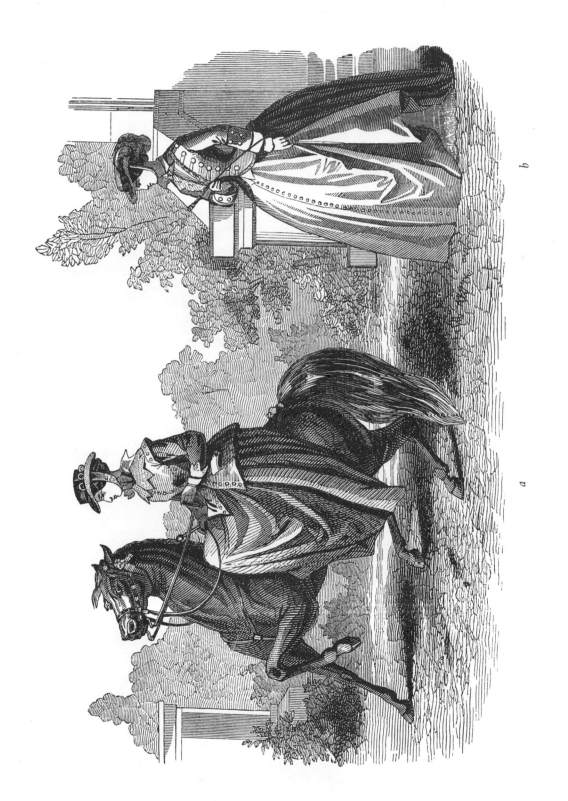

RIDING DRESSES. *Fig. a:* Habit of dark blue cloth; beaver hat. *Fig. b:* Mauve-colored cloth jacket trimmed with braid; habit skirt and sleeves of cambric; black felt hat with plumes (6/58).

b

a

31

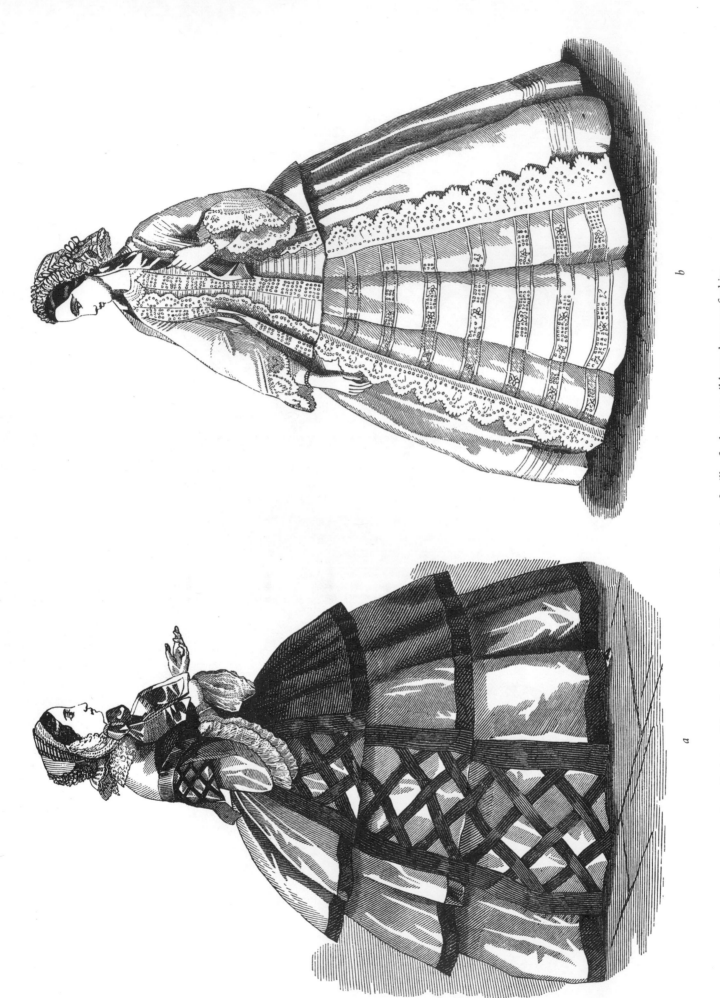

Fig. a: Lady's walking dress of peach-blossom silk; trimming of quills of pale-green ribbons; bonnet of white chip (6/58). *Fig. b:* Morning dress of fine French cambric; front arranged *en tablier;* cap of muslin and Valenciennes with loops of black velvet ribbon (7/58).

a

b

32

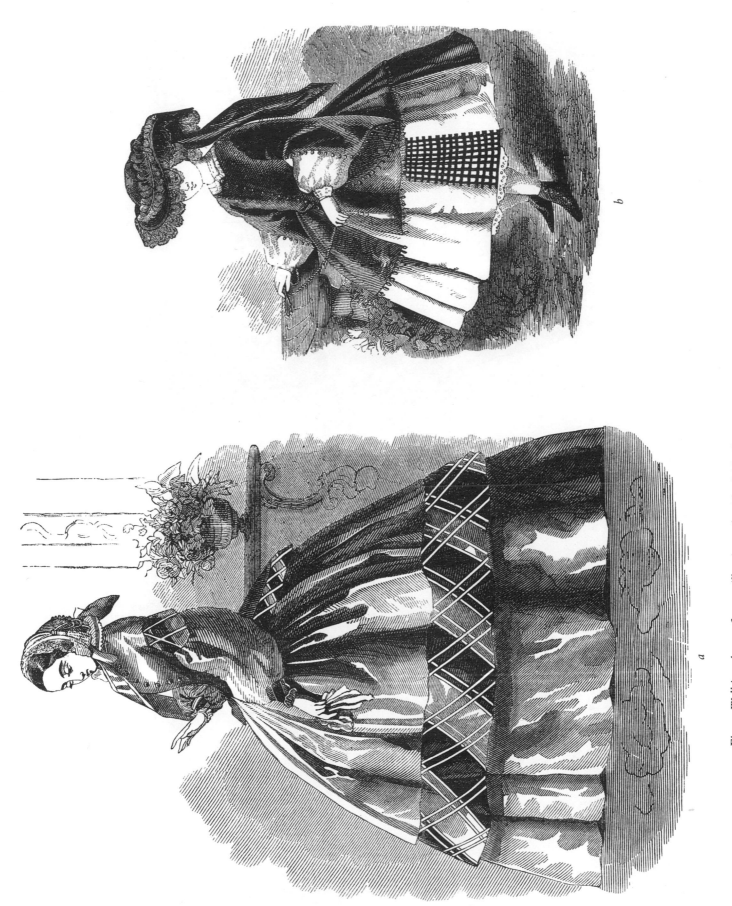

Fig. a: Walking dress of gray silk trimmed with plaid silk or velvet; corsage forms a vest in front and postillion jacket behind (7/58). *Fig. b:* Child's dress of pale lavender silk; checkerwork trimming of black velvet ribbon; street basque of black silk edged with *grelots* (8/58).

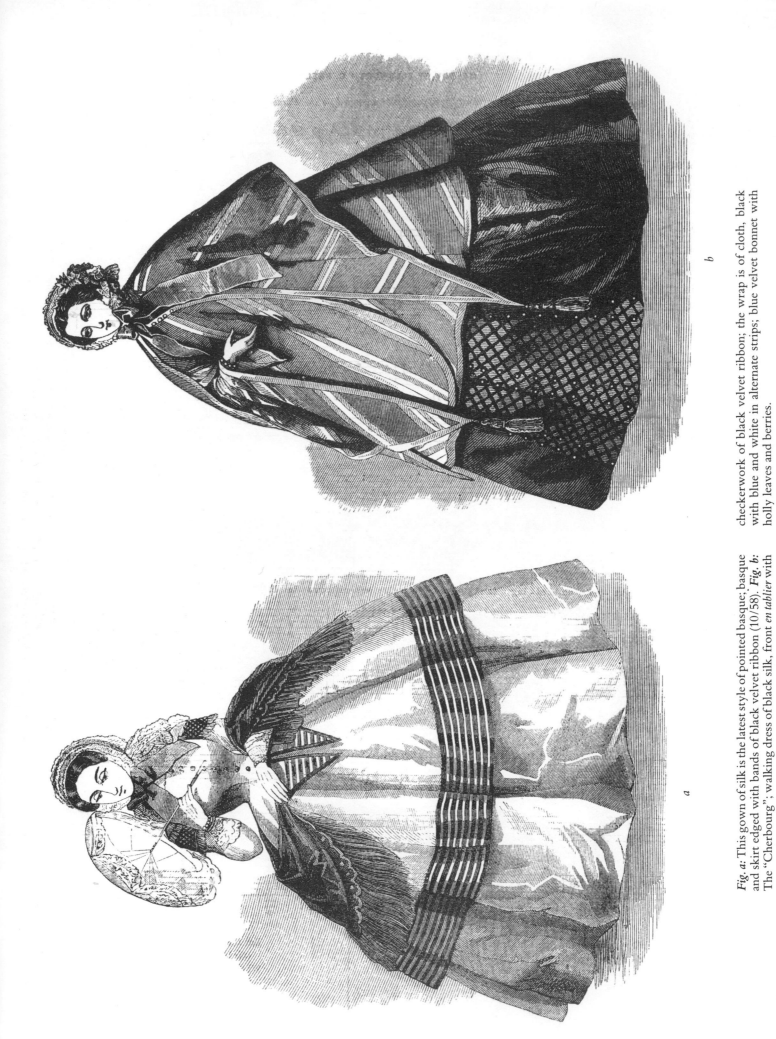

Fig. a: This gown of silk is the latest style of pointed basque; basque and skirt edged with bands of black velvet ribbon (10/58). *Fig. b*: The "Cherbourg", walking dress of black silk, front *en tablier* with checkerwork of black velvet ribbon; the wrap is of cloth, black with blue and white in alternate strips; blue velvet bonnet with holly leaves and berries.

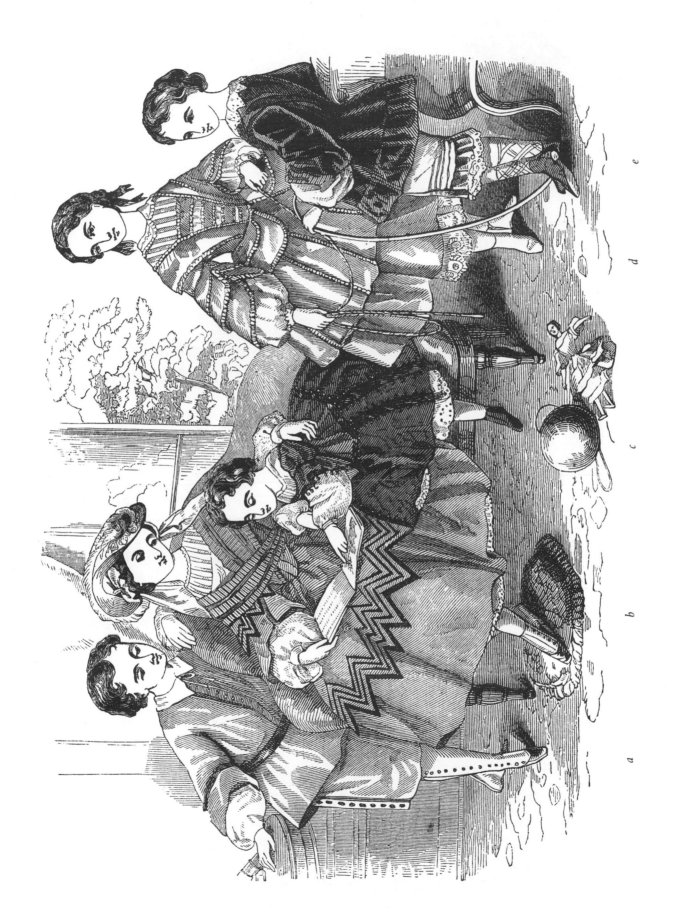

CHILDREN'S FASHIONS. *Fig. a:* Boy's sacque and trousers of garnet cashmere; collar and sleeves of cambric or linen. *Fig. b:* Party dress of lavender silk trimmed with black velvet ribbons; chemisette and sleeves of Swiss muslin. *Fig. c:* Dress of royal blue cashmere with trimming of velvet bands and *grelots*. *Fig. d:* Dress for a girl of twelve; green silk trimmed with quilling of ribbon. *Fig. e:* Boy's dress; blouse of royal purple velvet; white trousers. Dress suitable for a child's party.

a   b   c   d   e

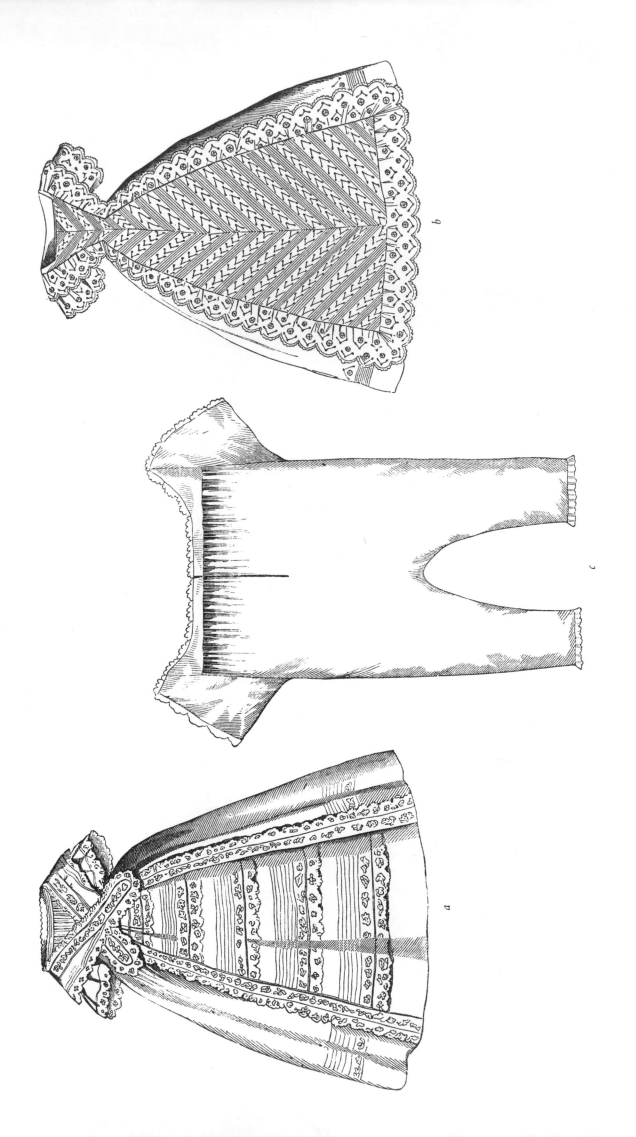

Fig. a: Christening robe made with *bretelles* and *tablier* front. *Fig. b:* Infant's robe of *broderie Anglaise;* broad *tablier* front; chemisette top (12/58). *Fig. c:* "The Nonpareil garment," combining the chemise and drawers, has many advantages. It is recommended especially to ladies traveling, to those giving out their wash, and to ladies boarding. It is also decidedly cooler for summer (8/58).

36

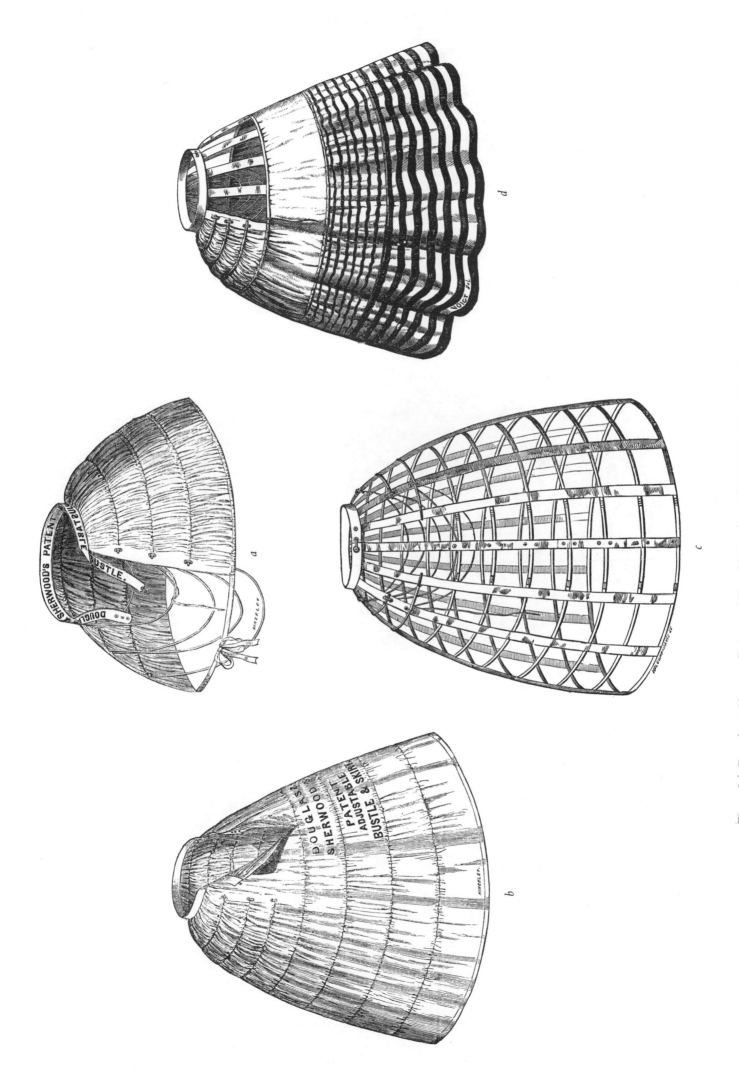

Figs. a & b: Douglas & Sherwood's Patent Adjustable Bustle and Skirt (2/58). *Fig. c*: Douglas & Sherwood's New Expansion Skirt (5/58). *Fig. d*: Douglas & Sherwood's Patent Balmoral Skirt (7/58).

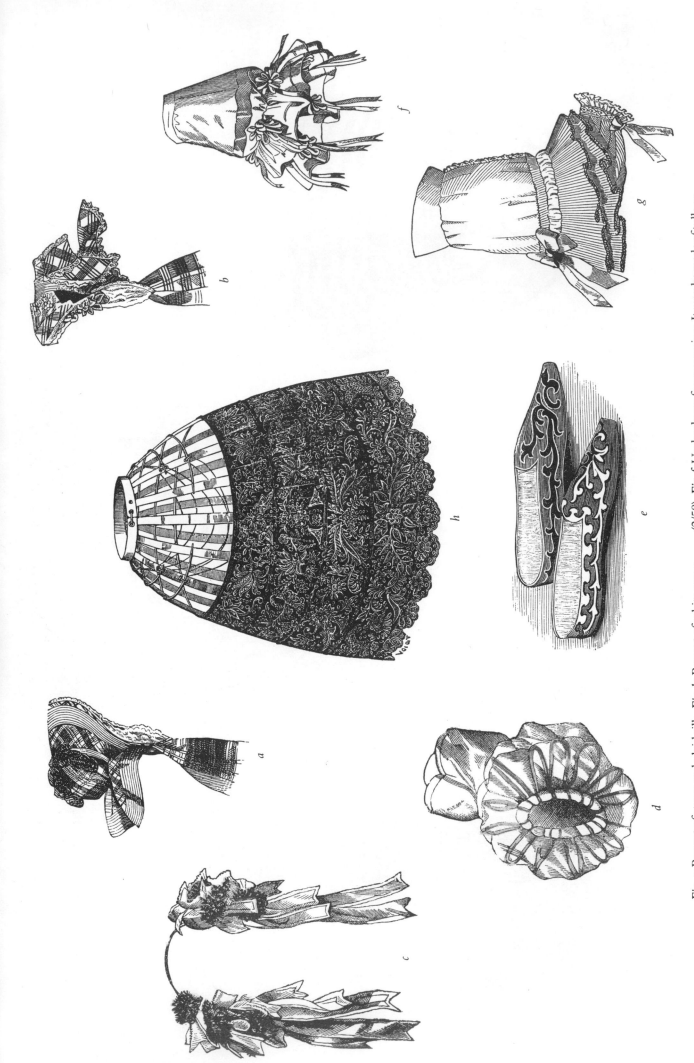

Fig. a: Bonnet of straw and plaid silk. *Fig. b*: Bonnet of white crape with bands of very bright plaid; trimmed with blonde lace; inside trimming of scarlet velvet ribbon and scarlet and white flowers (9/58). *Fig. c*: Headdress of ribbon mingled with tufts of fine flowers. *Fig. d*: Puffed undersleeve of tulle or muslin with narrow blue ribbon lacings (4/58). *Fig. e*: Slippers trimmed with appliqués (2/58). *Fig. f*: Undersleeve for mourning. It may be made of tulle or lace with knots of violet-colored satin ribbons at intervals. *Fig. g*: Mourning sleeve with double quilled band of lace or muslin (if black, in crape) (12/58). *Fig. h*: The Honiton Skirt, with the adjustable bustle (11/58).

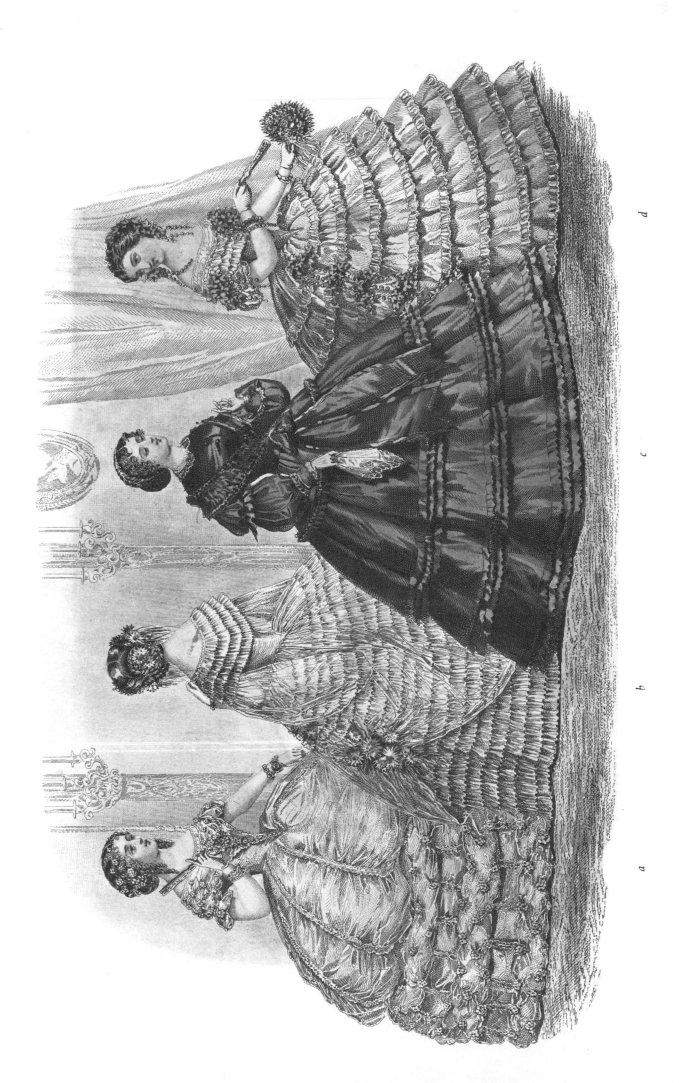

DRESSES FOR A PARTY. *Fig. a:* White silk dress covered with illusion and trimmed with ruching of blonde lace and blue flowers; wreath of forget-me-nots. *Fig. b:* Dress of white silk with seventeen fluted flounces; "angel" sleeves; overdress of illusion caught up with bright flowers and grass. *Fig. c:* Dress of violet silk trimmed with pinked ruffles, the center being green; headdress of violet chenille net and black velvet. *Fig. d:* "Tarietane" dress flounced over silk; bertha at neckline; rose-colored flowers trim dress and form headdress (9/60).

39

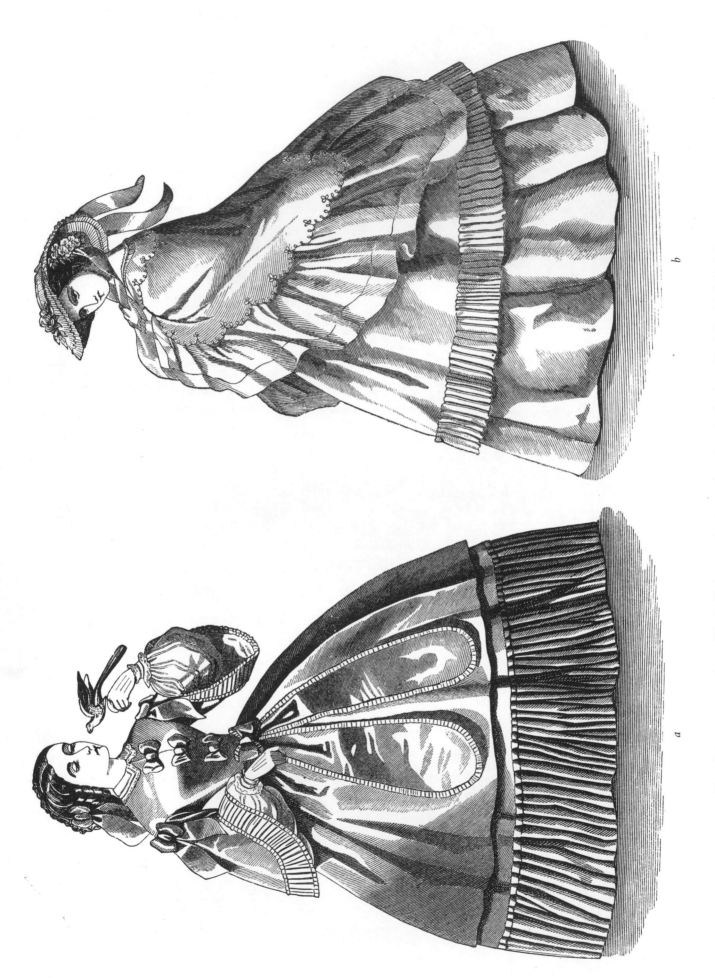

Fig. a: Dinner or street dress of black silk; bows and sash are of purple *moire d'antique. Fig. b:* "La Mathilde"; a becoming and comfortable dress for the country or a watering place. It can be made of silk, cloth or a thin material (9/60).

b

a

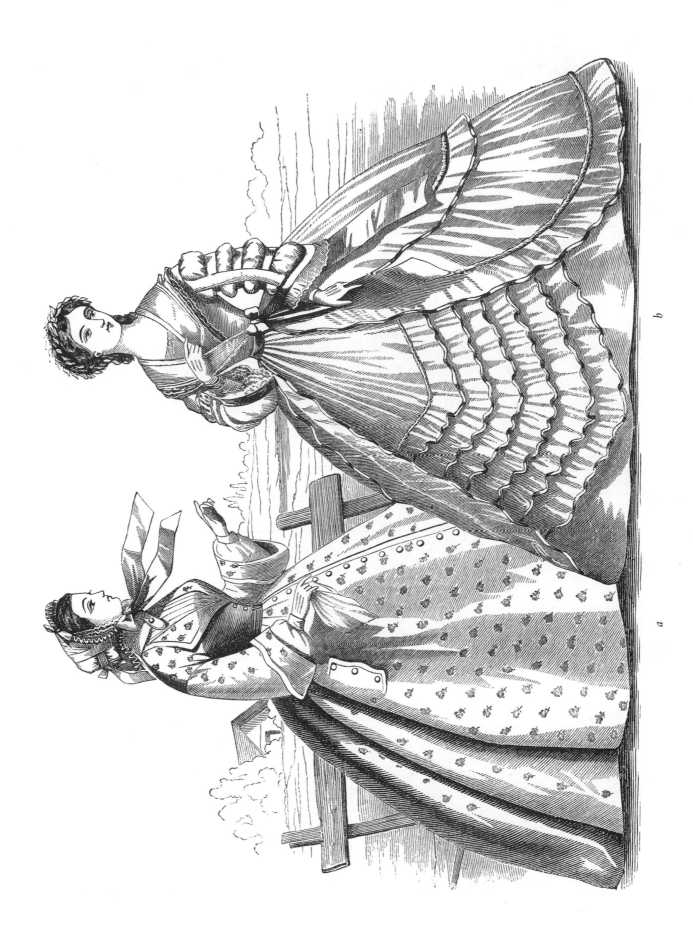

Fig. a: Outdoor dress for the country; robe of white piqué sprigged with small bouquets in brown and pink; edgings of white braid; bonnet of straw with crown and curtain of black silk; trimmed with pink ribbon. *Fig. b:* Evening dress for the sea; dress of clear muslin over slip of green silk; belt and trimmings of green silk ribbons (9/60).

41

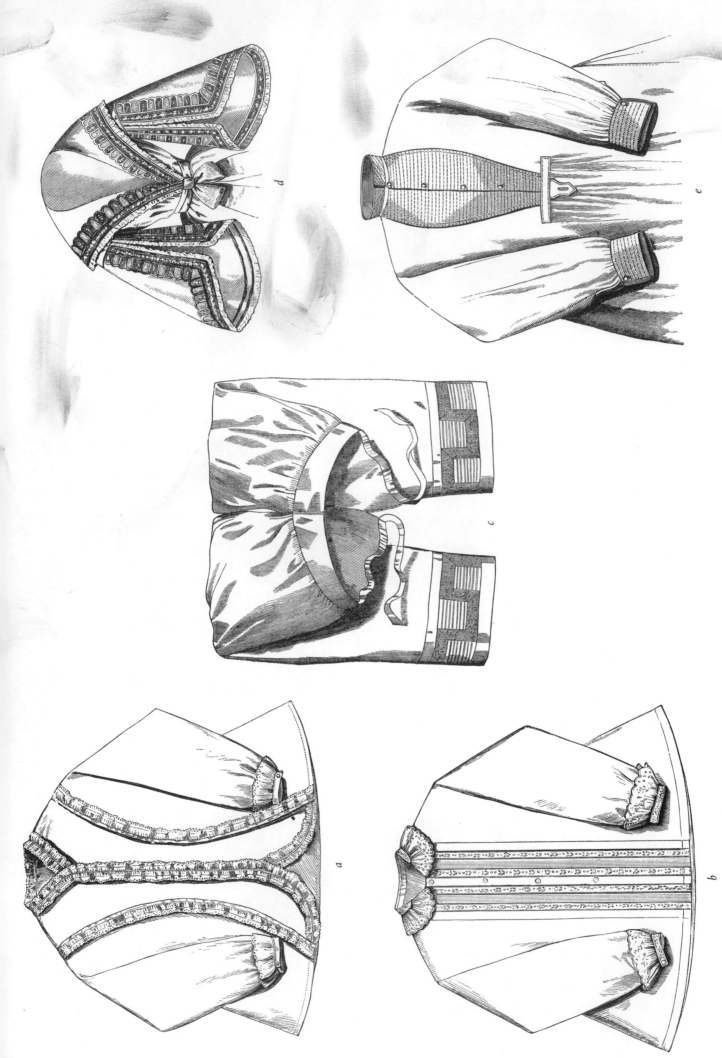

Figs. a & b: Ladies' short nightdresses (9/60). *Fig. c*: Ladies' drawers. *Fig. d*: Morning robe of white piqué with cape collar. *Fig. e*: Gentleman's shirt (5/61).

42

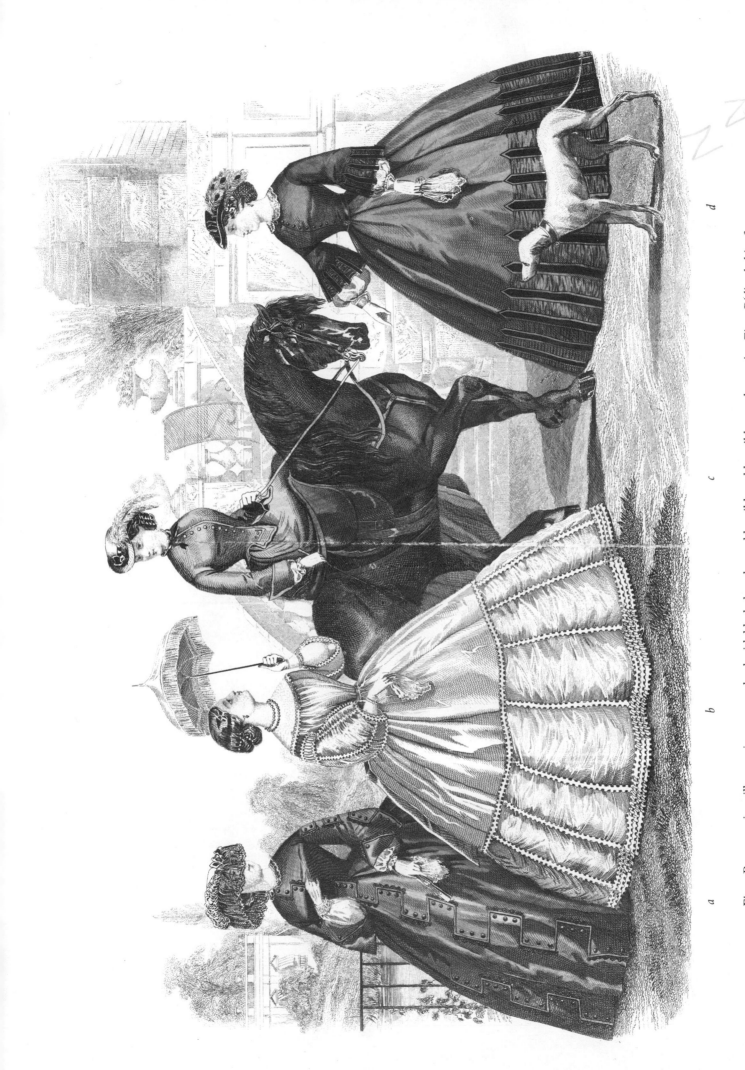

Fig. a: Brown spring silk one-piece gown edged with black thread lace; buttons of silk with velvet centers; English split straw hat. *Fig. b:* Dress (suitable for a watering place or evening company) of white *glacé* silk trimmed with *bouillonnés* or puffs of box-pleated blue ribbon; blue-ribbon sash at waist. *Fig. c:* Riding habit of green cloth; leghorn Spanish hat with white plume. *Fig. d:* Gown of purple silk with purple velvet trim; black straw hat with peacock plumes (5/61).

43

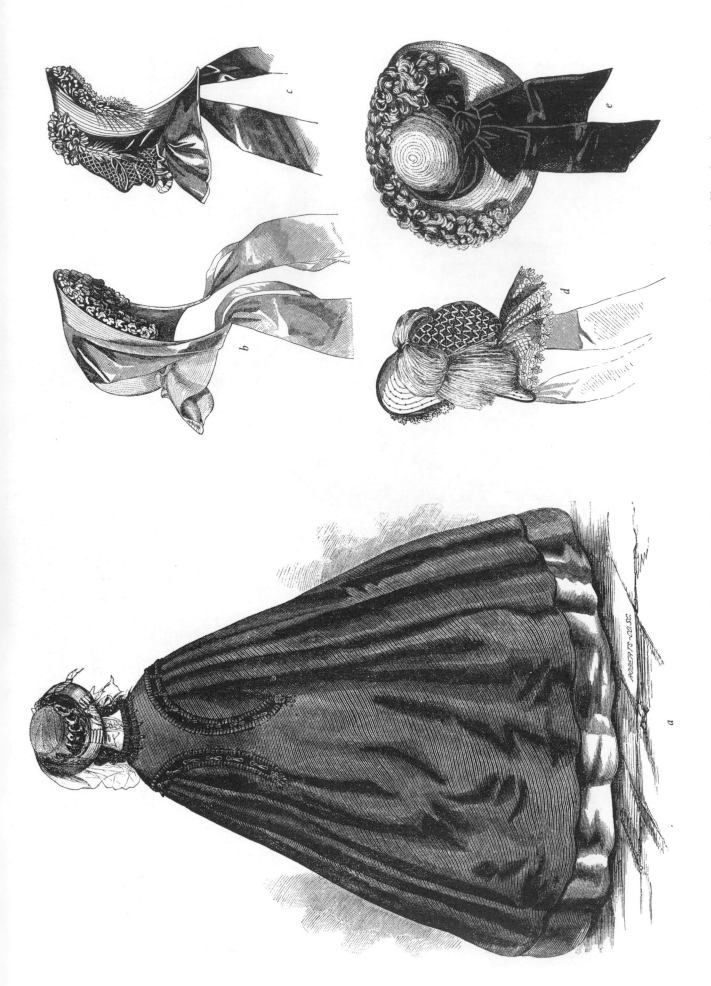

Fig. a: "The Aragonese"; a mantle of black taffeta trimmed with a passementerie with a ruched edge. *Fig. b:* Leghorn bonnet with wide green ribbon with a large bunch of violets on left side; faced with violet crape. *Fig. c:* Leghorn bonnet trimmed with black ribbon and scarlet flowers; cape and front of bonnet bound in scarlet velvet. *Fig. d:* Fancy straw bonnet with edge of front bound in black velvet; trimmed with bunches of yellow grass; black lace over maize–colored silk cape and strings. *Fig. e:* Brown leghorn straw hat with full brown feather and black velvet ribbon (7/61).

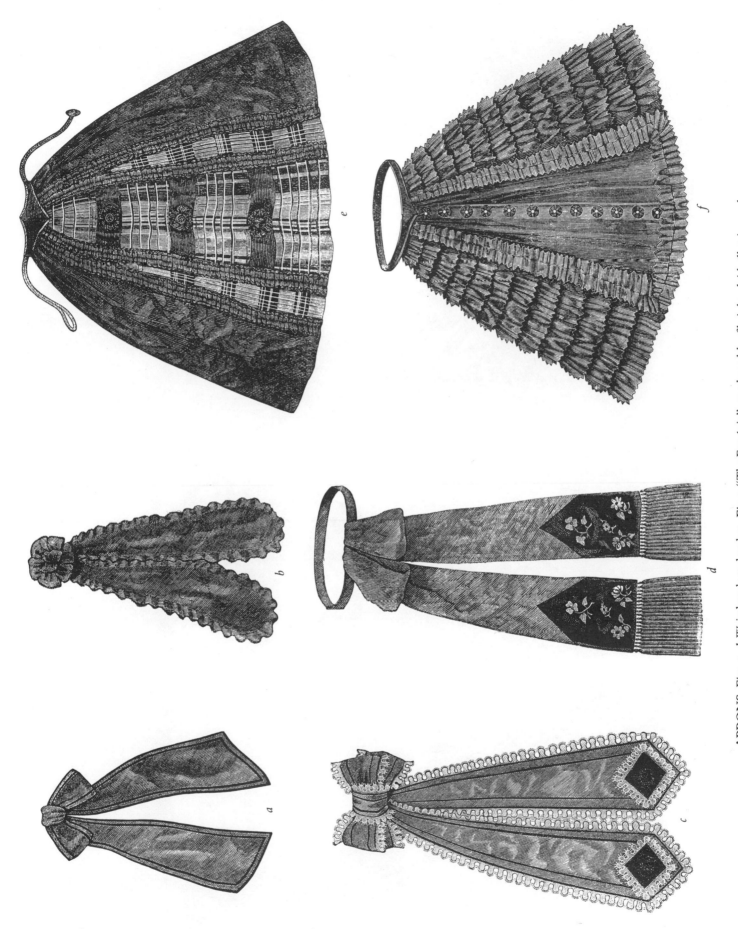

APRONS. *Figs. a–d:* Waistbands and sashes. *Fig. e:* "The Eugénie"; one breadth of bright plaid silk trimmed with lace and quilled ribbon; black *moire d'antique* on each side. *Fig. f:* "The Pompadour"; groseille silk trimmed with pink ruffles and quilling; velvet buttons down center (7/61).

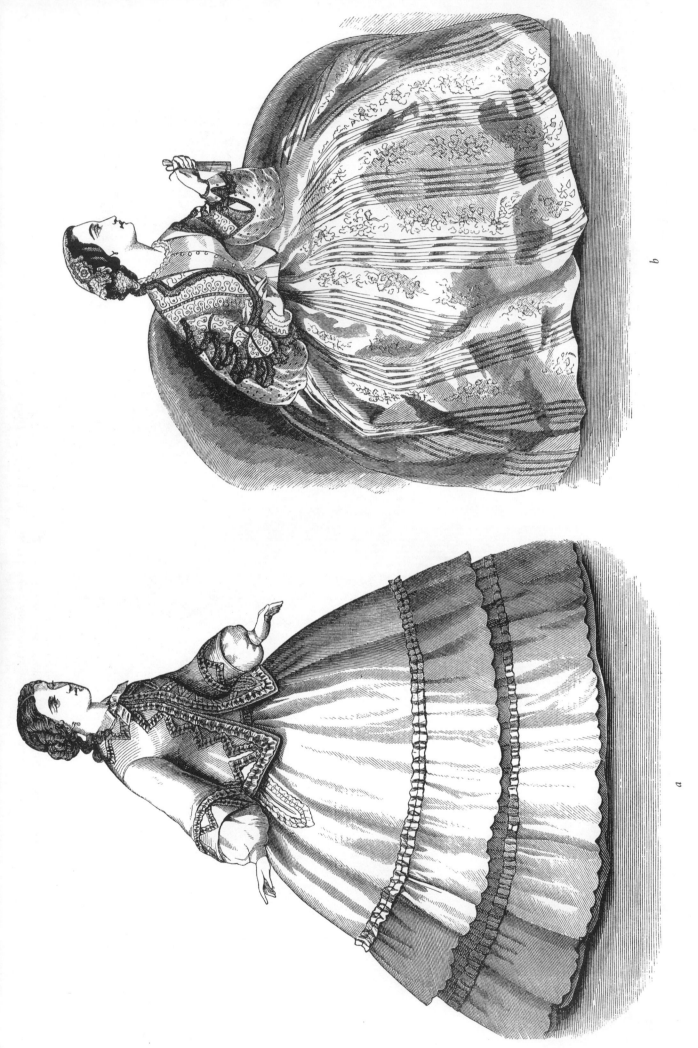

Fig. a: "The Imperial Jacket"; violet silk skirt with ruches in a darker shade; jacket of black silk trimmed with violet (7/62). *Fig. b:* "The Clarenda"; an organdy skirt; fancy Zouave braided with black and trimmed with black lace; white silk vest (11/62).

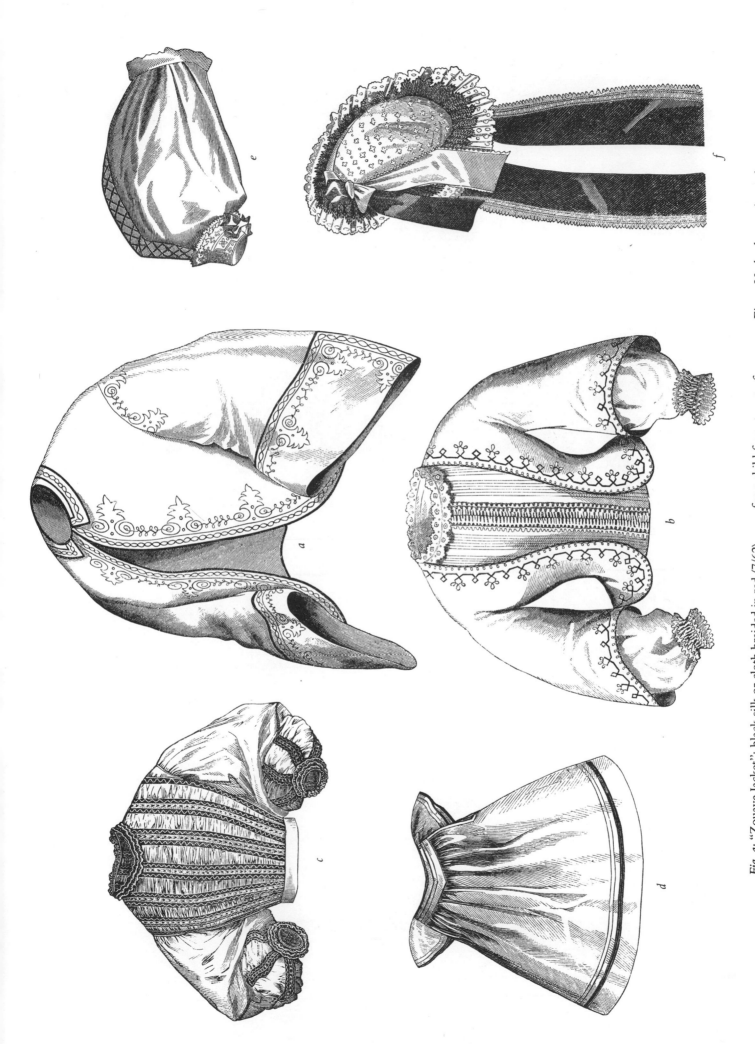

Fig. a: "Zouave Jacket"; black silk or cloth braided in red (7/62). *Fig. b:* Zouave jacket and Garibaldi shirt; of white piqué trimmed with black braid (8/62). *Fig. c:* White puffed spencer. *Fig. d:* Apron for a child from two to four years. *Fig. e:* Undersleeve trimmed with black velvet. *Fig. f:* Breakfast cap of figured muslin; trimmed with black lace and green and white ribbons (12/62).

47

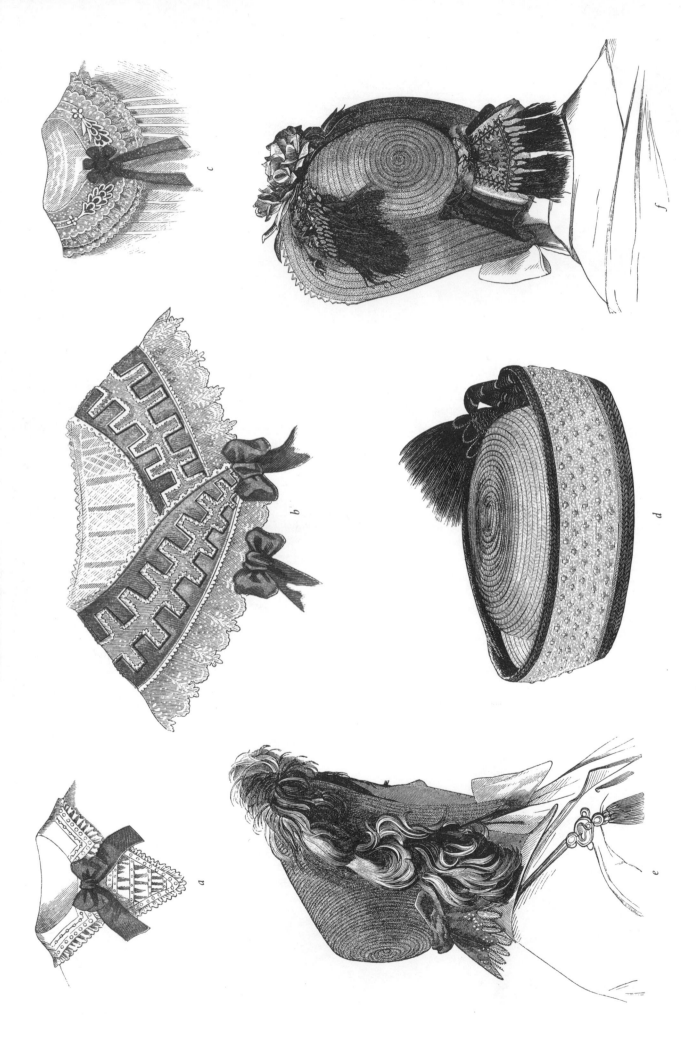

Fig. a: Linen collar and pointed chemisette trimmed with fluted ruffling (11/62). *Fig. b:* Fichu *Impératrice;* blue silk with embroidered muslin inserts; pattern defined by narrow dark ribbon; trimmed with point lace. *Fig. c:* Fancy muslin collar trimmed with Valenciennes lace. *Fig. d:* "Tudor Hat" of felt, velvet or all kinds of straw (7/62). *Fig. e:* Light gray straw hat trimmed with gray feathers; gray silk cape with fall of black lace. *Fig. f:* Chip straw bonnet trimmed with pink roses and a barbe of black lace embroidered with straw; fringed ends (8/62).

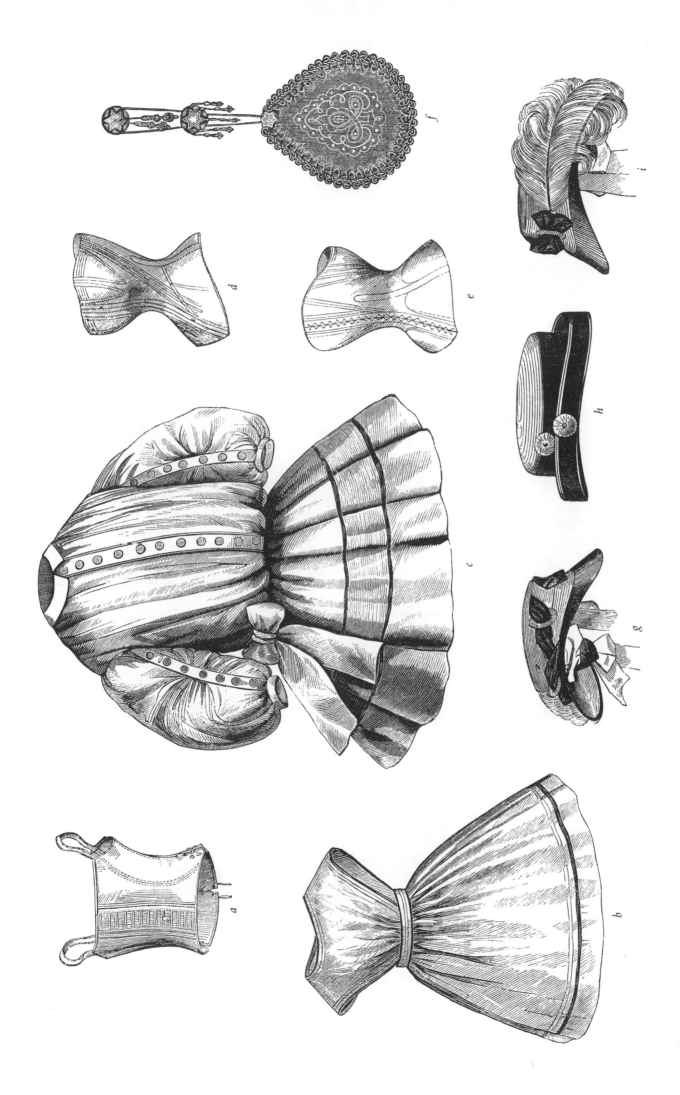

Fig. a: Corset for a little girl. *Fig. b:* School apron for a little girl. *Fig. c:* Little girl's "High Garibaldi Costume"; this costume could be made of any summer material; sash worn with the costume generally worn on the right. *Figs. d & e:* Madame Demorest's new French corset. *Fig. f:* Embroidered chatelaine of purple velvet trimmed with gold bullion, purple and gold gimp, embroidered in yellow floss with passementerie cords and tassels. *Fig. g:* Hat of gray straw resembling boy's cap trimmed with velvet flowers and a plume. *Fig. h:* Another view of the hat. *Fig. i:* "The Irving Hat" (7/62).

49

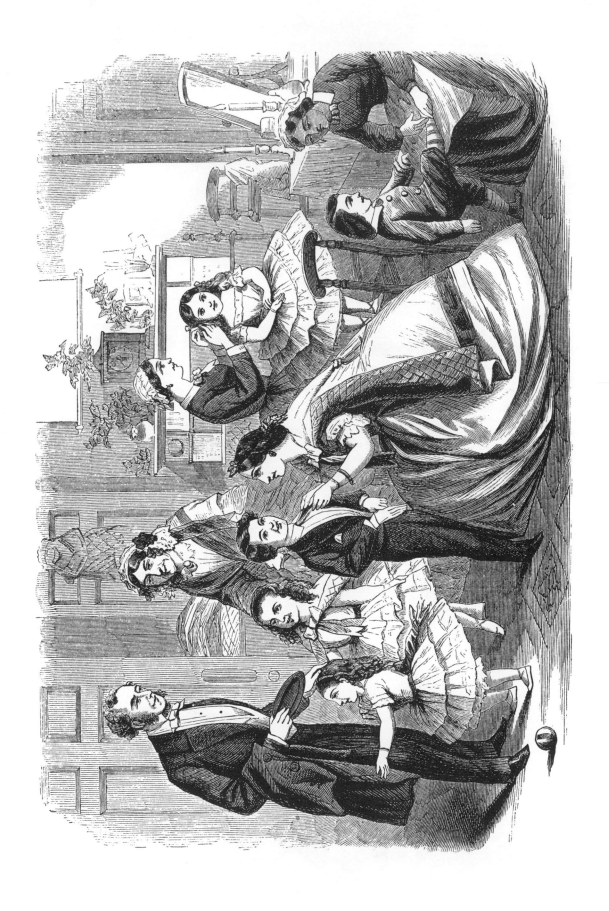

"Preparing for the Christmas Party" (12/62).

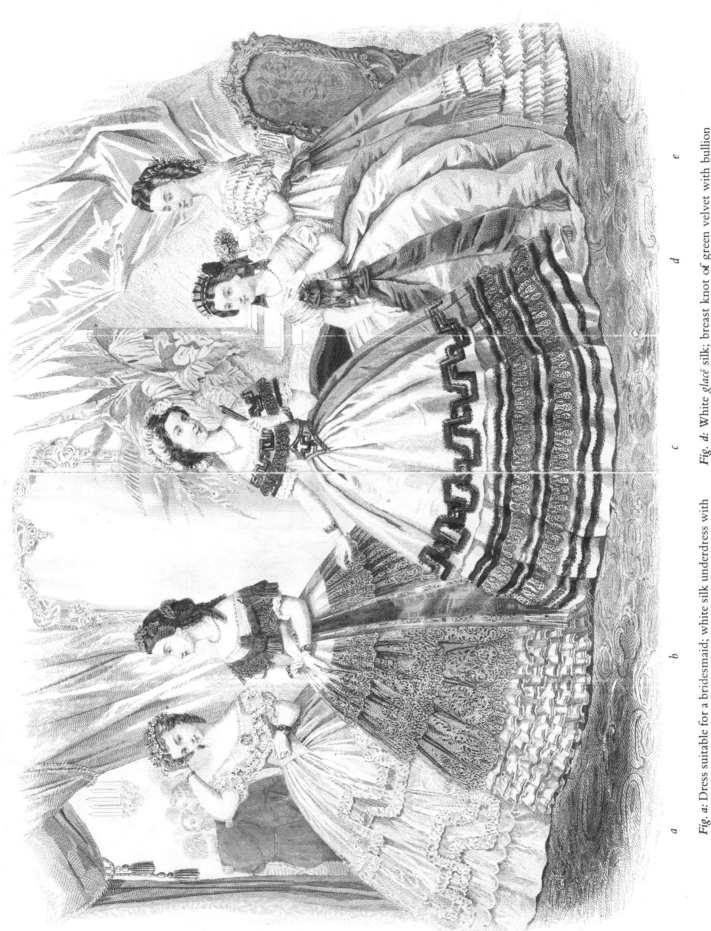

a　　　　b　　　　c　　　　d　　　　e

Fig. a: Dress suitable for a bridesmaid; white silk underdress with overdress of white crape; Etruscan ornaments; coiffure of cherries with foliage. *Fig. b:* Dress of white crape trimmed with viclet; skirt has three black thread lace flounces; coiffure of Parma violets. *Fig. c:* White satin dress trimmed with groseille velvet and black lace.

Fig. d: White *glacé* silk; breast knot of green velvet with bullion tassels; sash of green velvet finished with heavy bullion tassels. *Fig. e:* Dress suitable for a bridesmaid, of white muslin with gauffered flounces around hem; heavily fringed pink sash (1/63).

51

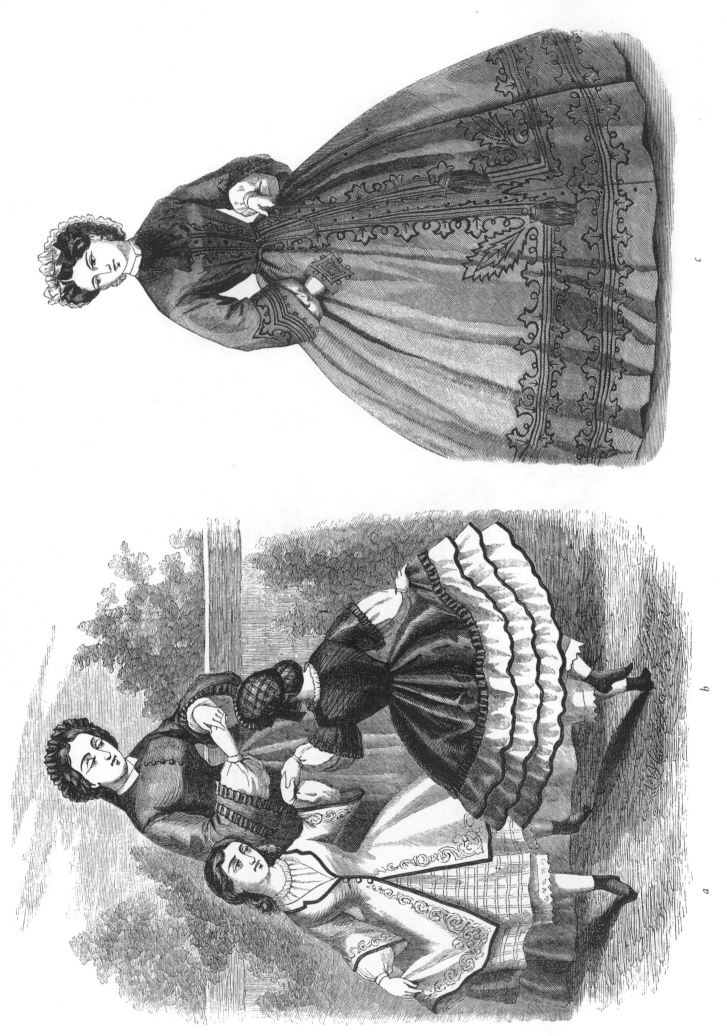

Figs. a & b: Little girls' dresses. *Fig. c:* "The Soutache Robe"; alpaca with border of brown printed to imitate a rich braiding (5/63).

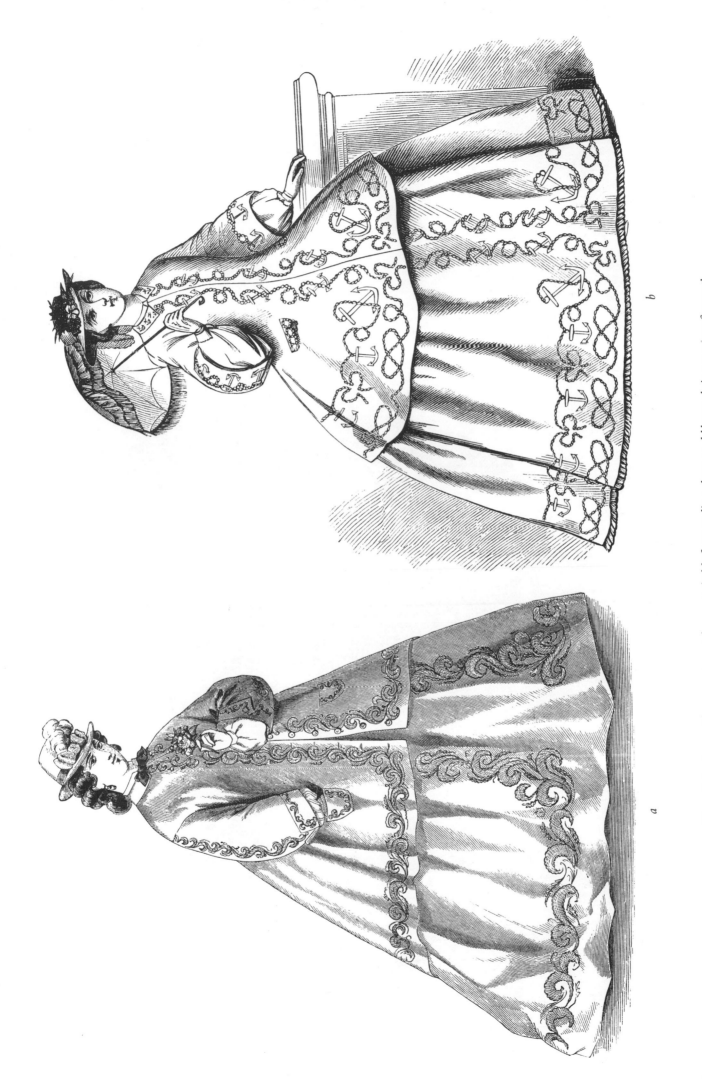

Fig. a: Robe dress with sacque to match, very suitable for traveling; dress could be made in percales of neutral tints or in taffeta or alpacas (6/63). *Fig. b:* Fancy paletot for the country; costume could be made of wool or silk and either mohair or silk can be used for the braiding (7/63).

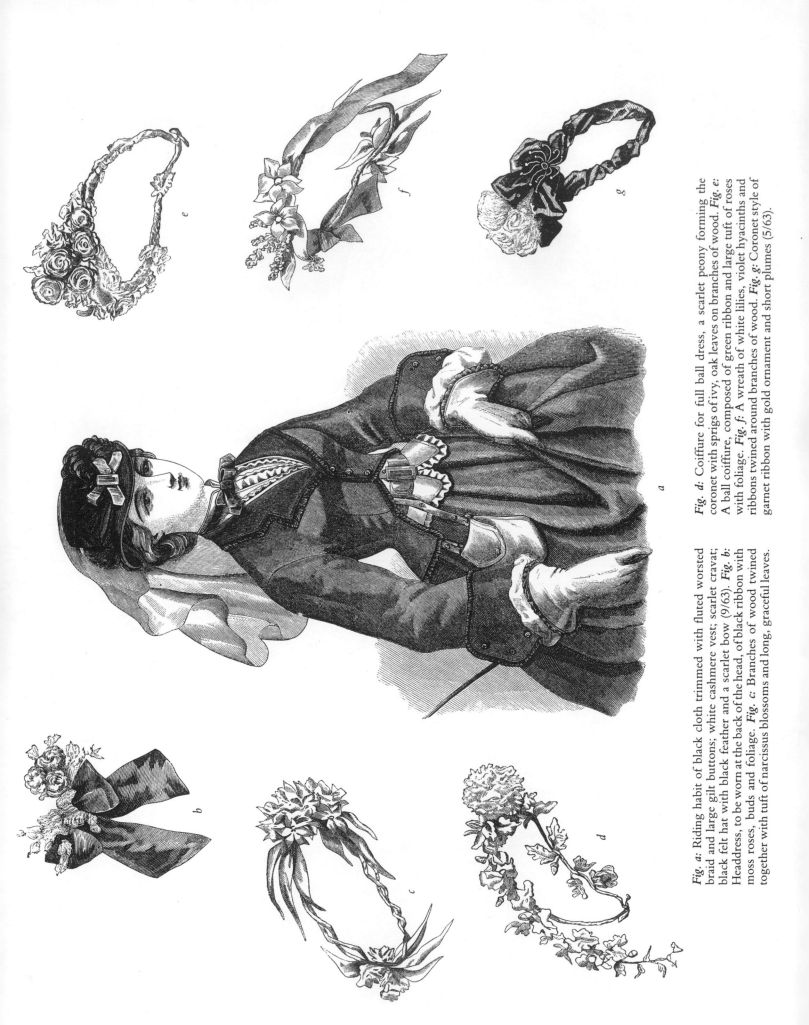

Fig. a: Riding habit of black cloth trimmed with fluted worsted braid and large gilt buttons; white cashmere vest; scarlet cravat; black felt hat with black feather and a scarlet bow (9/63). *Fig. b:* Headdress, to be worn at the back of the head, of black ribbon with moss roses, buds and foliage. *Fig. c:* Branches of wood twined together with tuft of narcissus blossoms and long, graceful leaves. *Fig. d:* Coiffure for full ball dress, a scarlet peony forming the coronet with sprigs of ivy, oak leaves on branches of wood. *Fig. e:* A ball coiffure, composed of green ribbon and large tuft of roses with foliage. *Fig. f:* A wreath of white lilies, violet hyacinths and ribbons twined around branches of wood. *Fig. g:* Coronet style of garnet ribbon with gold ornament and short plumes (5/63).

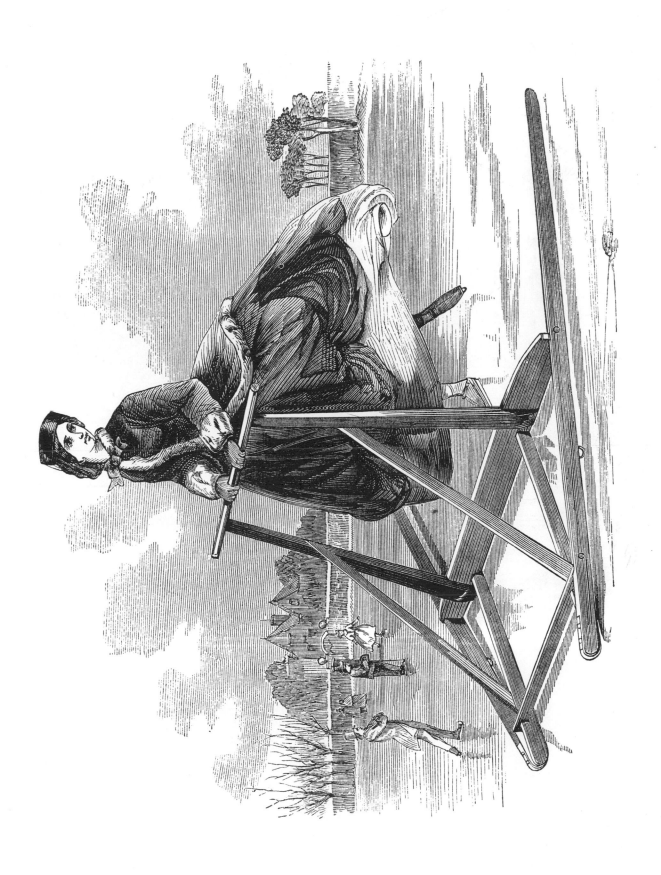

Skating costume (12/63).

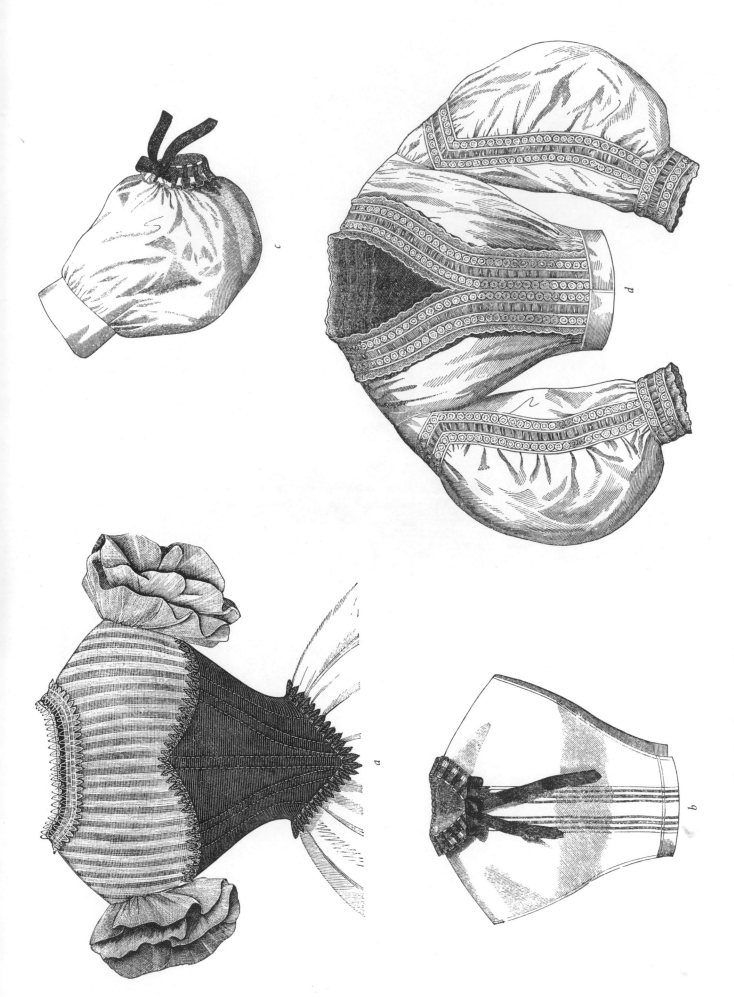

Fig. a: French corsage of black silk trimmed with guipure lace worn over a fine French muslin waist (10/63). *Figs. b & c*: Matching vestee and sleeves of muslin with slits with ribbon run through (1/63). *Fig. d*: Fancy spencer with puffings, insertions and lace (12/63).

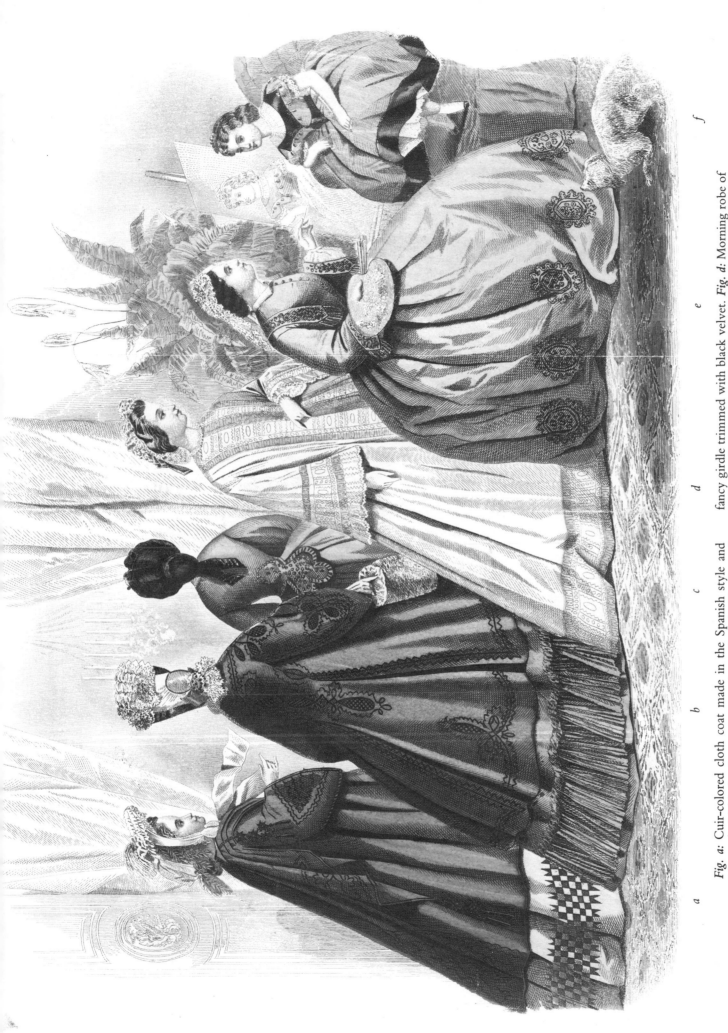

Fig. a: Cuir-colored cloth coat made in the Spanish style and trimmed with black velvet, worn over dress of purple silk trimmed with black velvet; white uncut velvet bonnet with falling crown of purple velvet trimmed with fern leaves. *Fig. b:* Cloak of black cloth trimmed with gimp ornaments; green silk dress with a deep chenille flounce; bonnet of white silk. *Fig. c:* Blue poplin dress with fancy girdle trimmed with black velvet. *Fig. d:* Morning robe of white muslin over dress of rose-colored silk; pink ribbon trim. *Fig. e:* Dress of light-colored cuir poplin trimmed with medallions of black velvet and braid; coiffure of white lace with magenta flowers. *Fig. f:* Child's dress of magenta silk poplin with a broad band of black velvet (1/64).

57

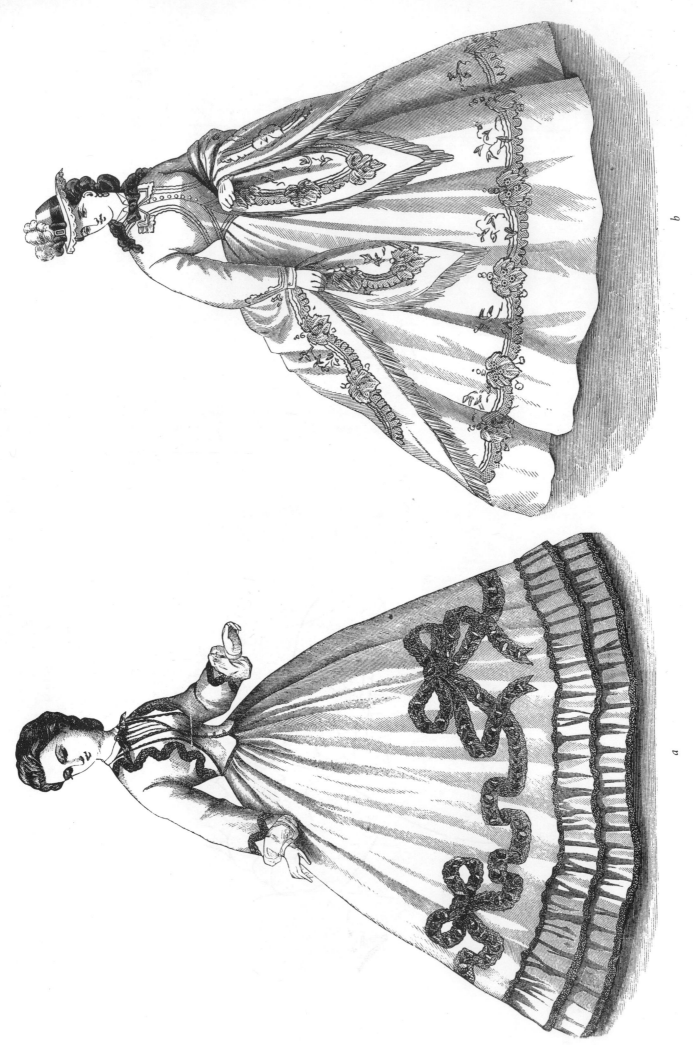

Fig. a: Visiting or dinner dress of sea-green silk; hem flounces edged with black guipure lace; design on skirt and jacket is of black guipure laid on white ribbon (2/64). *Fig. b:* Summer suit of cuir-colored "Glacina" stamped in a lace design; matching shawl is fringed (6/64).

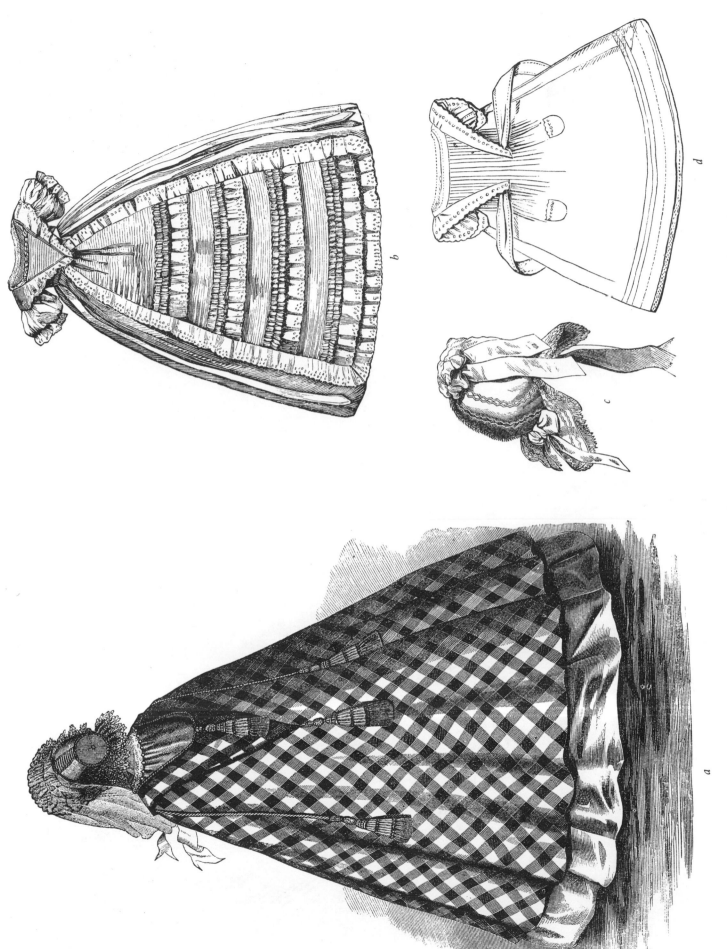

Fig. a: "The Hispania"; long cape with hood of bold plaid (5/64). *Fig. b:* Infant's robe. *Fig. c:* Infant's cap of white merino trimmed with white ribbons. *Fig. d:* Child's apron-dress (1/64).

59

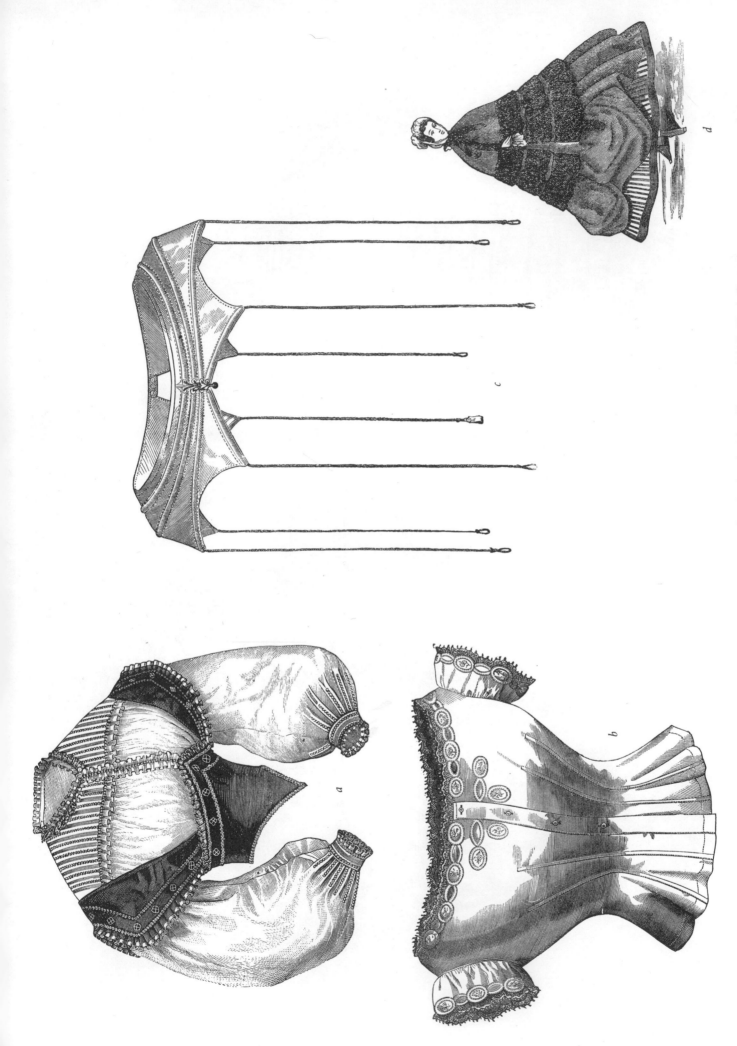

Fig. a: A bretelle corselet made of black velvet trimmed with white braid and buttons (4/64). *Fig. b:* Corset cover of fine cambric muslin trimmed with worked medallions and Valenciennes lace (5/64). *Fig. c:* The Pompadour porte-jupe, or dress elevator. *Fig. d:* The porte-jupe in use (6/64).

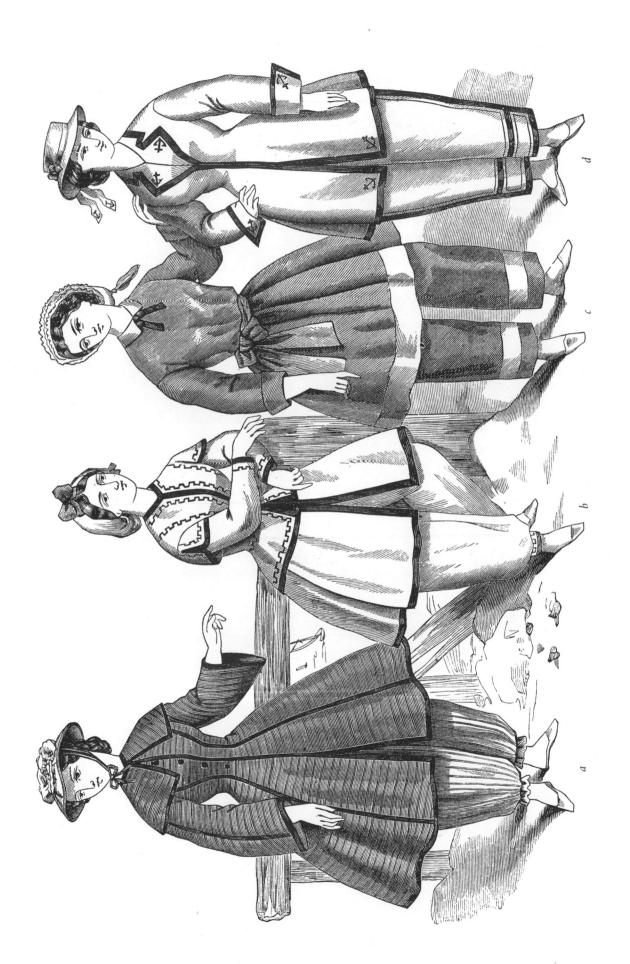

BATHING DRESSES. *Fig. a:* Turkish pants of gray-and-white–striped material fastened at ankle with elastic cord. Paletot dress of dark blue and black flannel edged in black; oil-silk hat with scarlet binding. *Fig. b:* Suit of pearl-colored flannel trimmed with dark blue flannel; cap of oil-silk trimmed with dark blue flannel. *Fig. c:* Suit of black cloth bound in scarlet flannel; cap trimmed with black braid and a long black tassel. *Fig. d:* Suit of scarlet flannel trimmed with bands of black braid; hat is straw with scarlet braid (7/64).

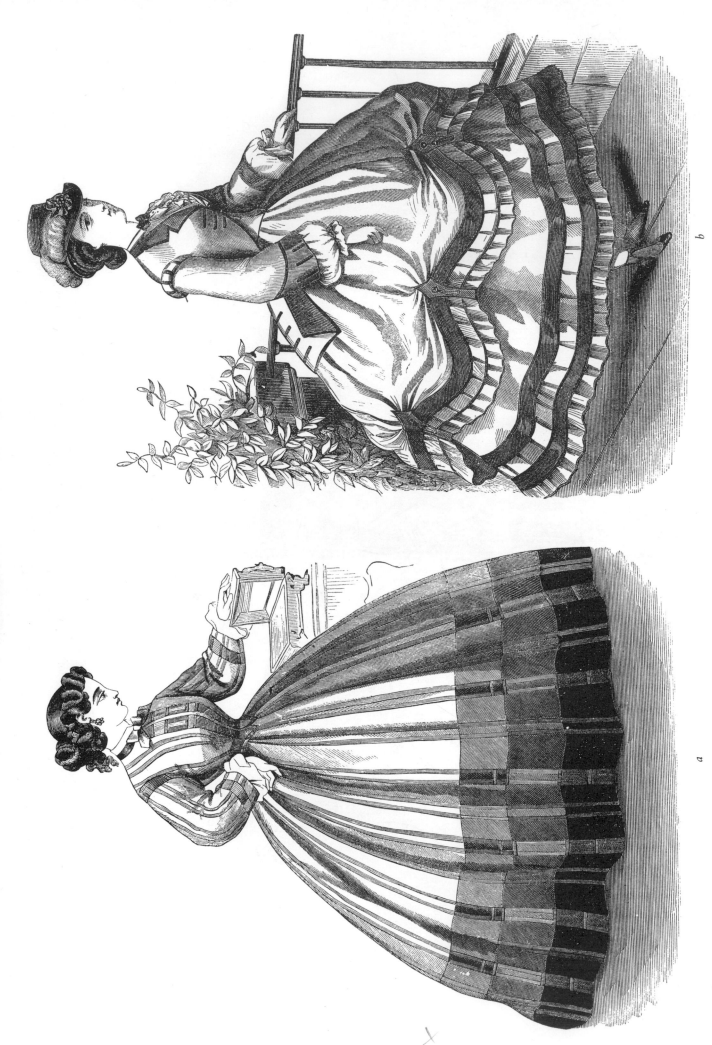

Fig. a: Organdy robe of rich salmon striped with chocolate brown; edge of skirt in different shades of brown (7/64). *Fig. b:* Dress for the seaside of buff alpaca; edge of skirt and overskirt jacket has bands of black velvet; postillion hat of black straw with velvet feather (8/64).

62

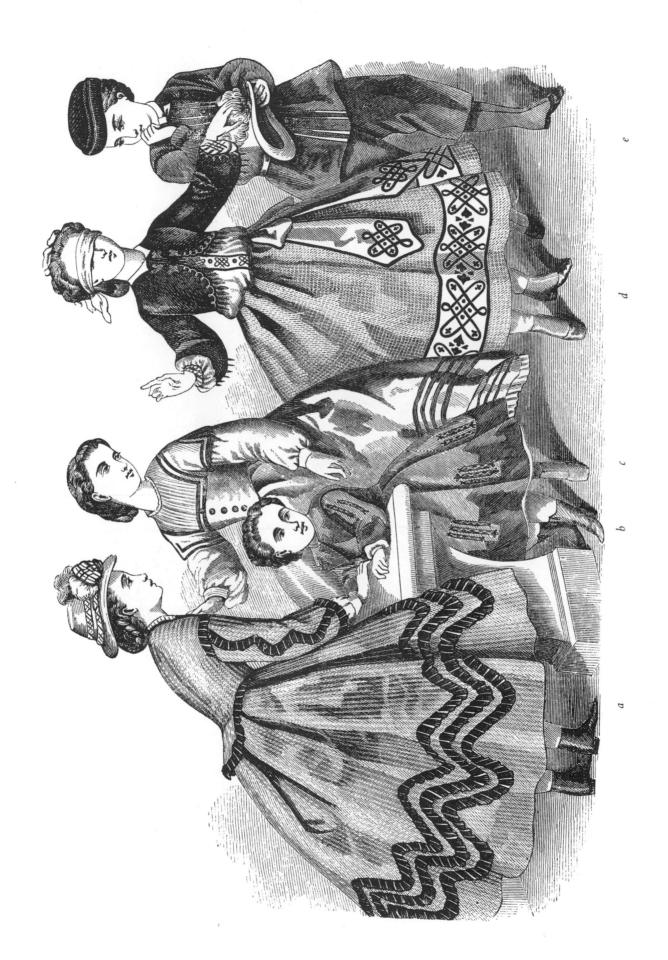

CHILDREN'S COSTUMES. *Fig. a:* Gray poplin dress with fluted ribbon of Tartan colors. *Fig. b:* Solferino merino dress with black-and-solferino-braid trim. *Fig. c:* Napoleon-blue cashmere dress trimmed with rows of black velvet. *Fig. d:* Gray cashmere skirt trimmed with bias band of white cashmere edged and braided in scarlet; scarlet cloth jacket braided with white and trimmed with black drop buttons. *Fig. e:* Blouse, pants and gaiters of gray; blue silk tie and black velvet cap (9/64).

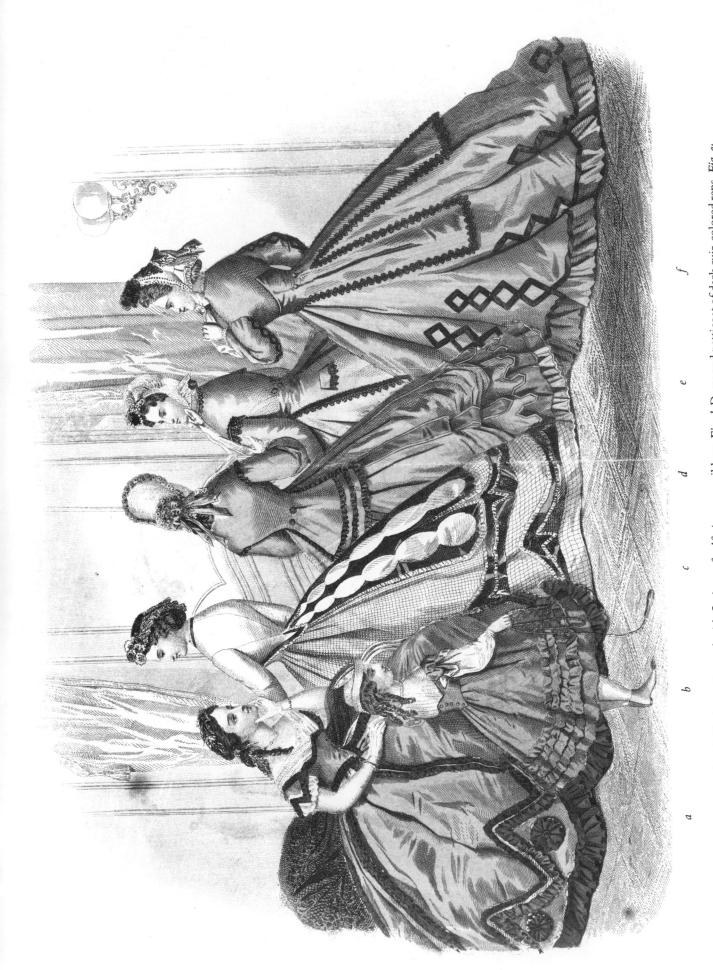

Fig. a: Fawn-colored silk dress trimmed with flutings of solferino silk. *Fig. b:* Child's dress of green silk with narrow pinked ruffles; corselet of green silk; white muslin gimp; white felt hat with white wing. *Fig. c:* Dinner dress of black-and-white crossbarred silk trimmed with applications of black velvet edged with white fluted ribbon. *Fig. d:* Dress and petticoat of dark cuir-colored reps. *Fig. e:* Visiting dress of pearl-colored lace; bonnet of white royal velvet with white feathers. *Fig. f:* Dress of purple silk edged with fluted ruffle and trimmed with black velvet; white bonnet with black lace, feathers and a large tuft of pink roses (12/64).

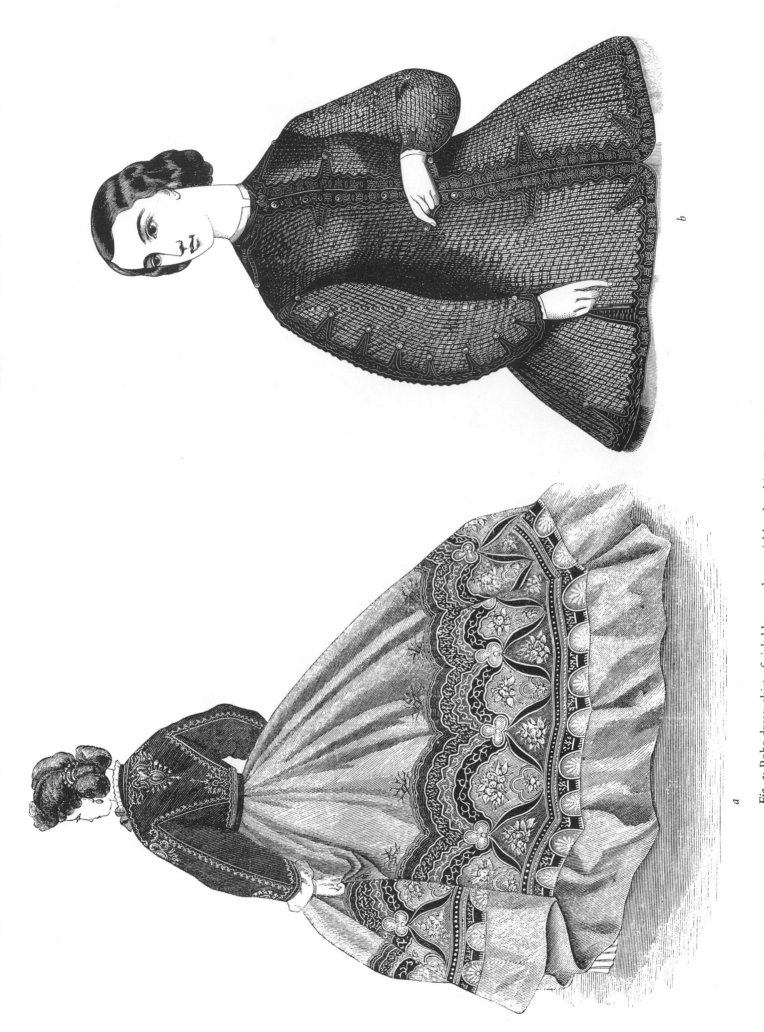

Fig. a: Robe dress; skirt of rich blue wool material bordered in a Persian design; Zouave of black wool material with patterns in bright colors (12/64). *Fig. b:* Winter jacket in double crochet (11/64).

65

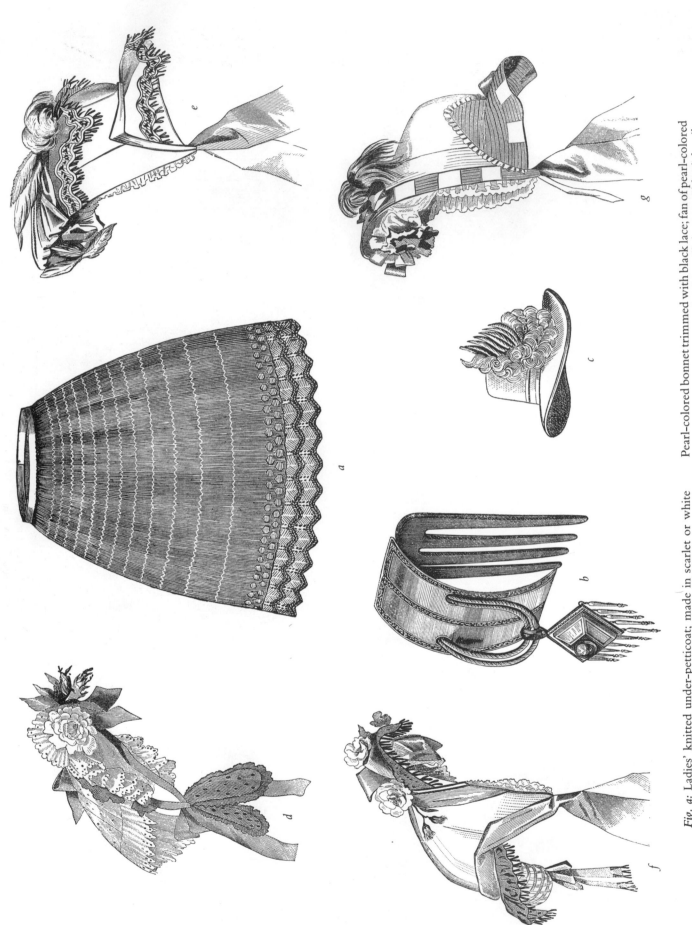

Fig. a: Ladies' knitted under-petticoat; made in scarlet or white wool (12/64). *Fig. b:* Fancy comb of gilt, elegantly ornamented with black enamel (9/64). *Fig. c:* Mousquetaire hat of drab straw with two narrow bands of scarlet velvet; plumes of black and red feathers and one large ostrich feather (7/64). *Fig. d:* Dinner cap of spotted tulle, trimmed with large pink rose and button. *Fig. e:*

Pearl-colored bonnet trimmed with black lace; fan of pearl-colored silk and white feathers. *Fig. f:* White silk bonnet with violet ribbons and pink roses; net formed of ribbons attached to bonnet. *Fig. g:* A leghorn bonnet trimmed with salmon and black ribbon; black feathers. Bonnet faced with scarlet velvet, black lace and salmon-colored flowers (9/64).

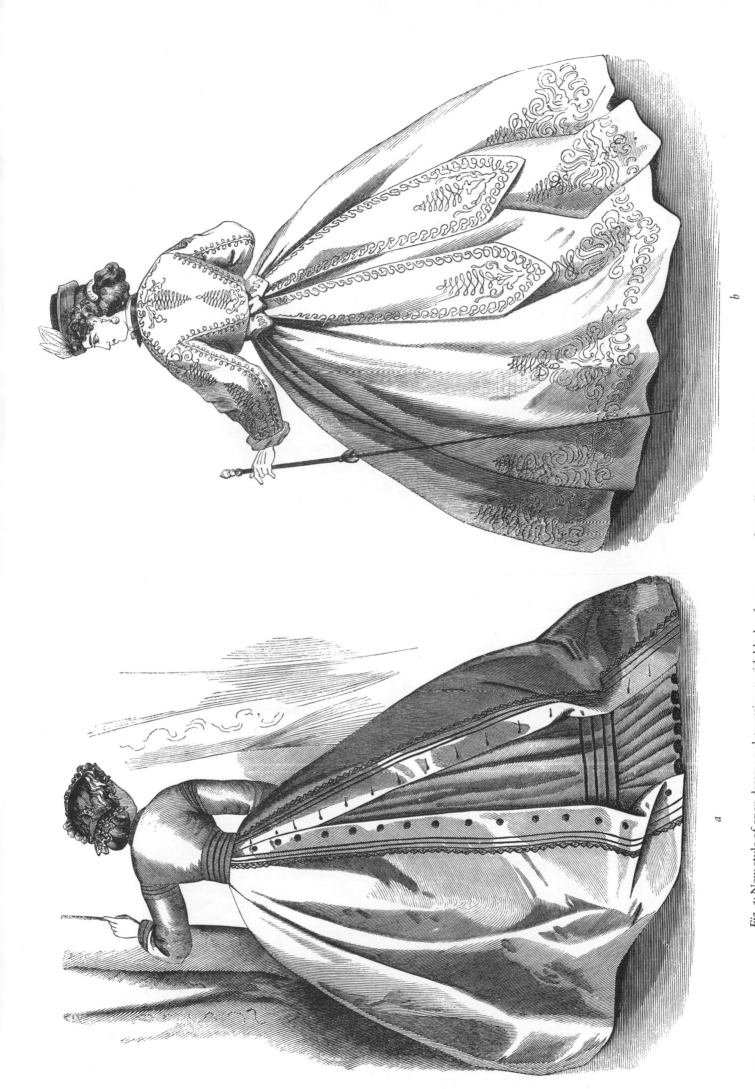

Fig. a: New style of open dress; scarlet petticoat with black velvet bands; dress of silver-gray poplin trimmed with black guipure lace, narrow black velvet and jet buttons; scarlet belt, collar, cuffs and epaulettes all trimmed with black velvet (3/65). *Fig. b:* Spring robe of pearl-colored cambric stamped to represent black braiding (4/65).

a

b

67

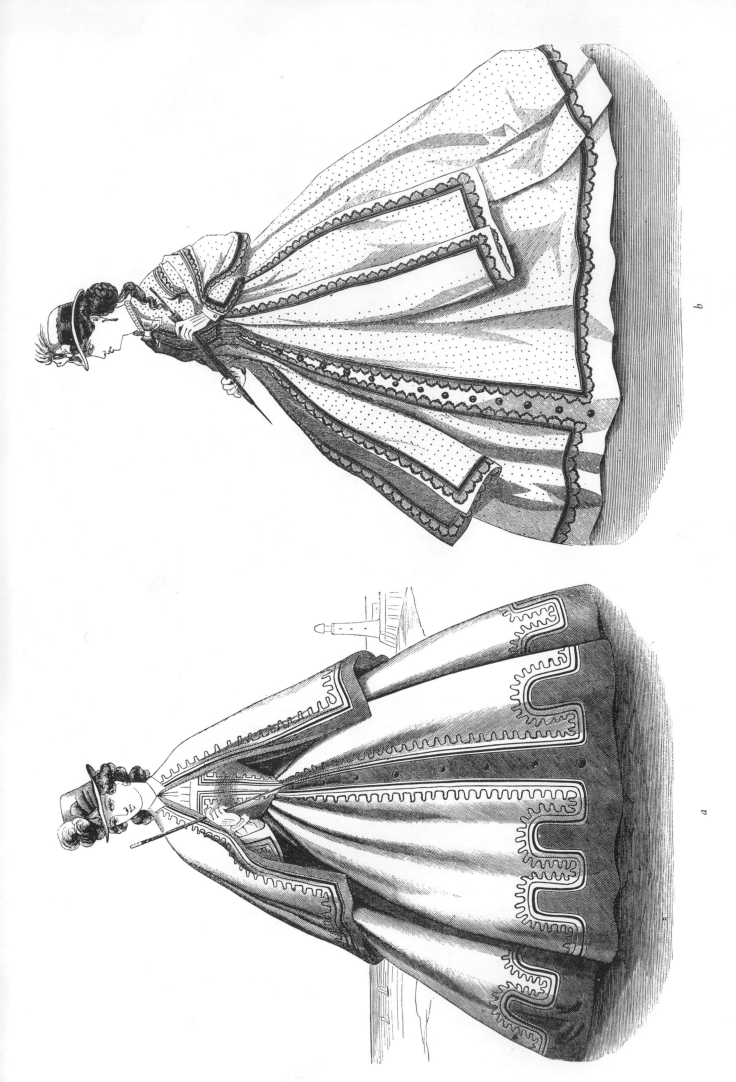

Fig. a: Robe Helvetienne; white cambric with bordering of delicate mauve outlined in black (5/65). *Fig. b:* Dress of white percale dotted with black and bordered with a lace design; matching scarf (7/65).

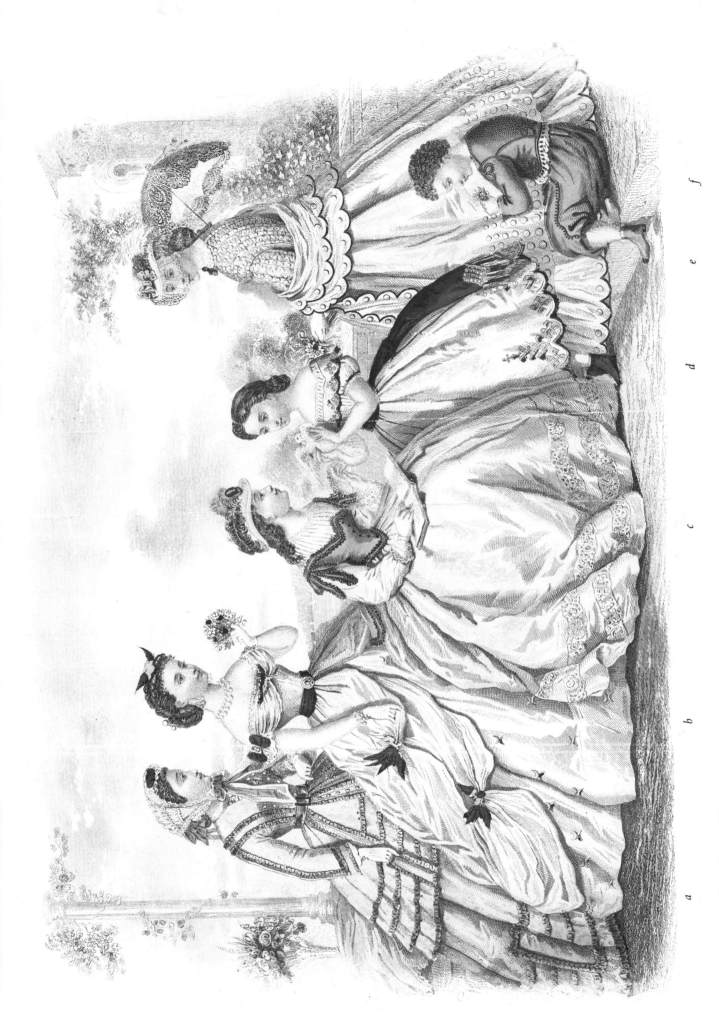

Fig. a: Dress of figured grenadine *barège* with fluted green-ribbon trim. *Fig. b:* Ball costume; underskirt of white silk embroidered with scarlet and blue crescents; upper skirt of white crape draped back by birds of brilliant plumage; scarlet velvet bows. *Fig. c:* Skirt of delicate shades of mauve goat's-hair cloth; fancy corsage of

purple silk; gimp and sleeves of French muslin. *Fig. d:* Dress of white alpaca, bound and braided with plum velvet; sash of plum-colored silk. *Fig. e:* Dress of white organdy, trimmed with black alpaca braid. *Fig. f:* Boy's Zouave suit of tan-colored summer cloth braided with silk cord and trimmed with drop buttons (8/65).

a   b   c   d   e   f

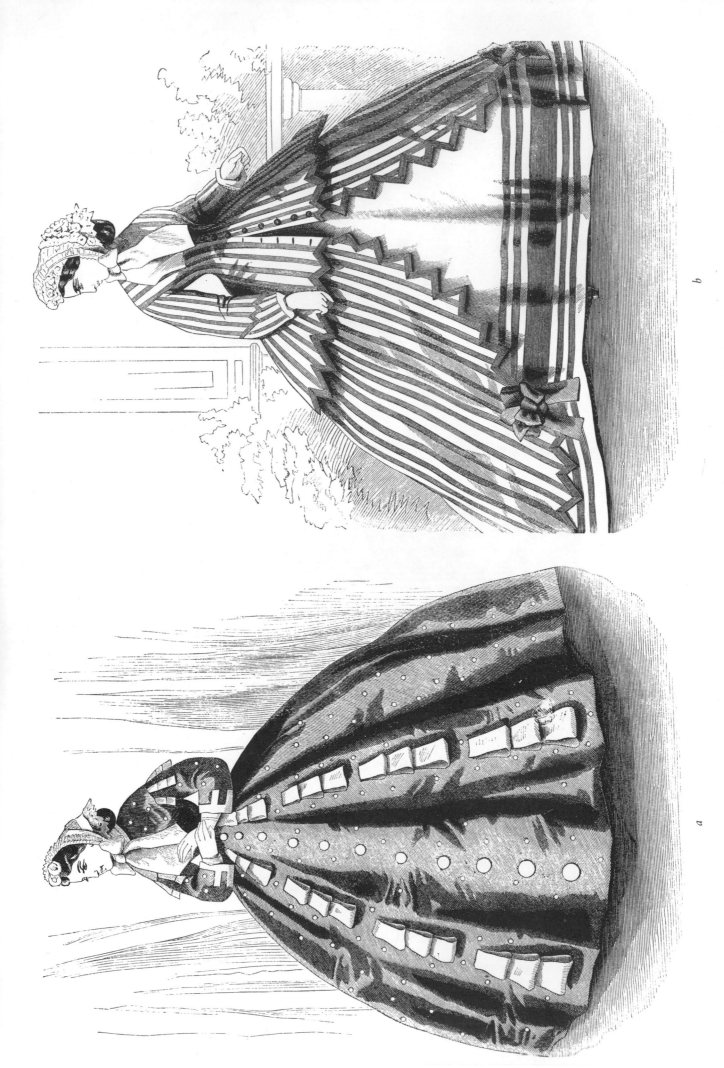

Fig. a: Walking dress of black foulard silk spotted with green; body and skirt trimmed with flat loops of green velvet ribbon (10/65). *Fig. b:* Costume for watering place; dress of blue-and-white-striped silk, made short and edged with points; underskirt of white with blue bands at hem (10/65).

b

a

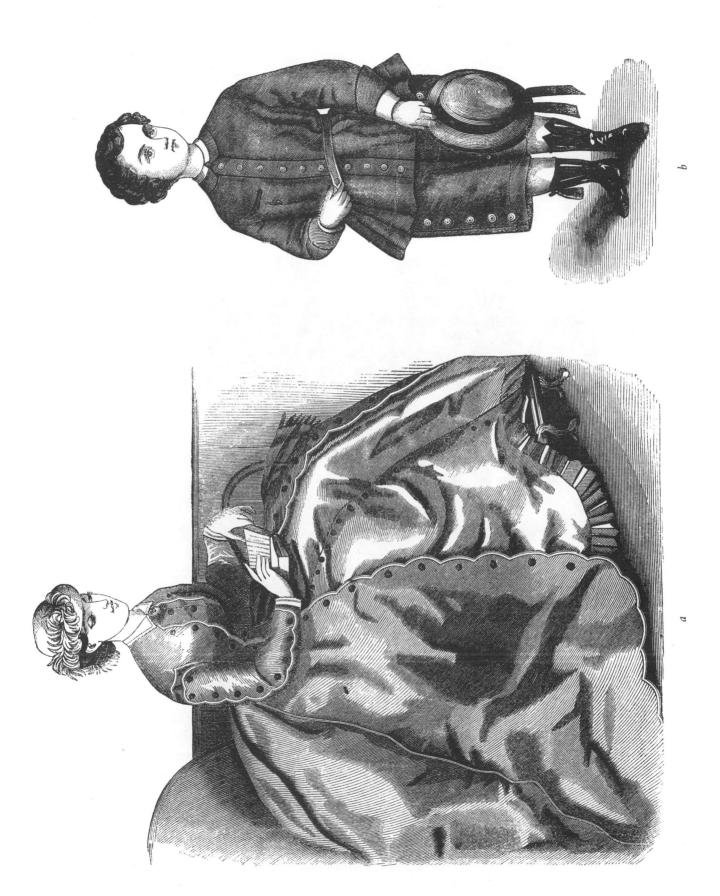

Fig. a: Visiting dress of lapis lazuli-colored poplin; scallops edged with white; buttons of black velvet (10/65).
Fig. b: Suit for boy from five to eight years old, of light gray cloth with mother-of-pearl buttons; gray straw hat with black ribbon; Polish boots with tassels (6/65).

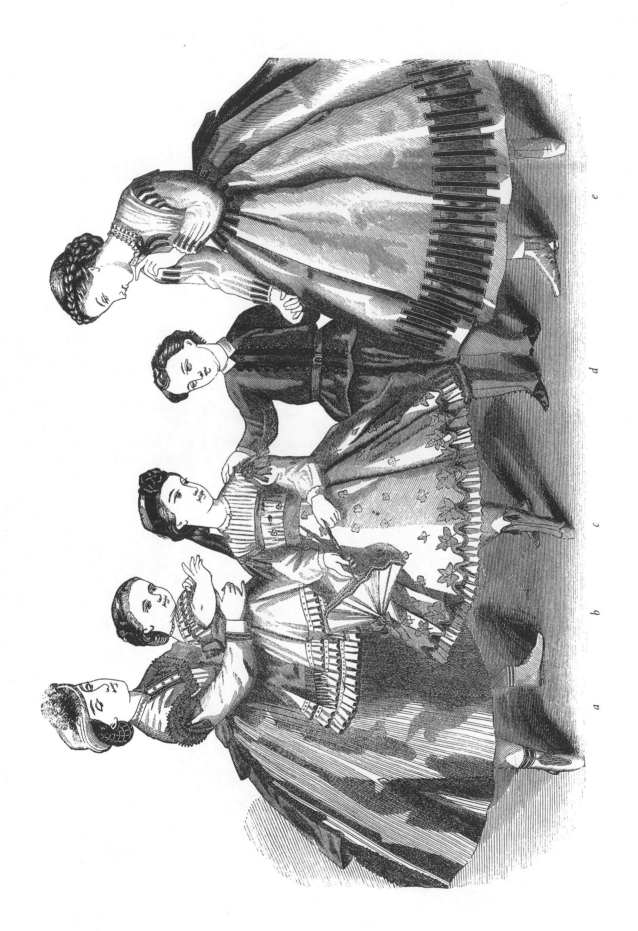

Fig. a: White striped alpaca dress trimmed with blue. *Fig. b*: Dress of French percale with a sash of rose-colored ribbon. *Fig. c*: Silk dress of gray sprigged with magenta; magenta leaves applied at hem. *Fig. d*: Boy's suit of light gray cloth. *Fig. e*: Skirt of light gray silk with wide bands of blue, striped with bands of black velvet at hem; waist is of white muslin, sash of black velvet (10/65).

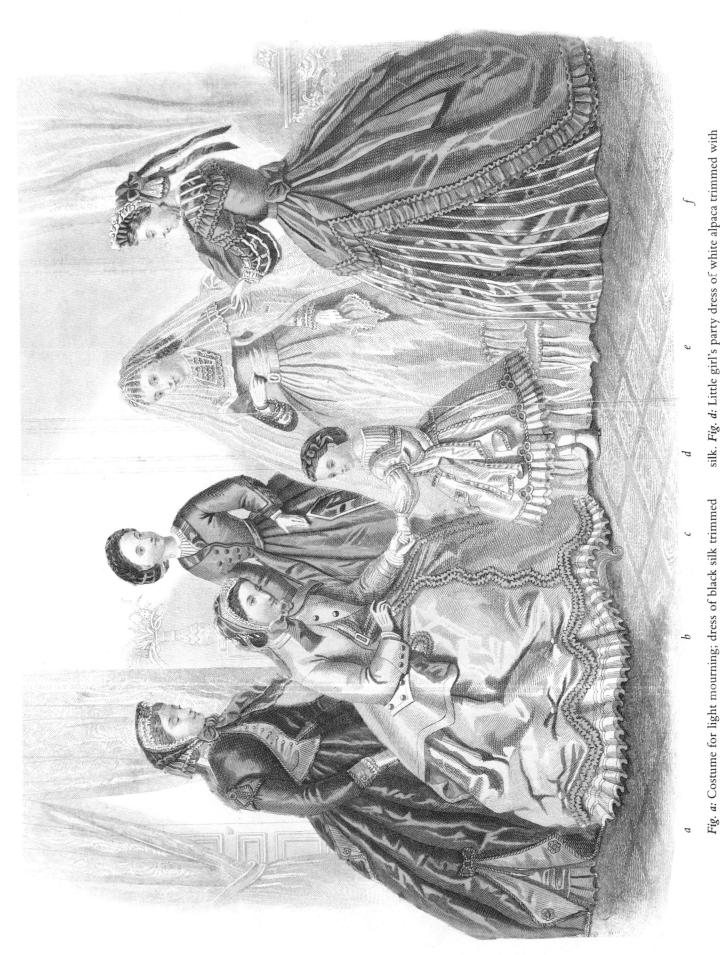

a b c d e f

Fig. a: Costume for light mourning; dress of black silk trimmed with thick cord and violet silk; front of corsage of violet silk. *Fig. b:* Walking costume; dress, paletot and petticoat of pearl-colored reps; trimmings and lining of paletot of violet silk. *Fig. c:* Dinner toilet; dress of coffee-colored poplin trimmed at bias with blue silk. *Fig. d:* Little girl's party dress of white alpaca trimmed with yellow ribbon and cords. *Fig. e:* Bridal toilet; dress of heavy white silk; corsage has rows of appliqué lace; tulle veil. *Fig. f:* Reception dress of blue silk and blue-and-white-striped silk.

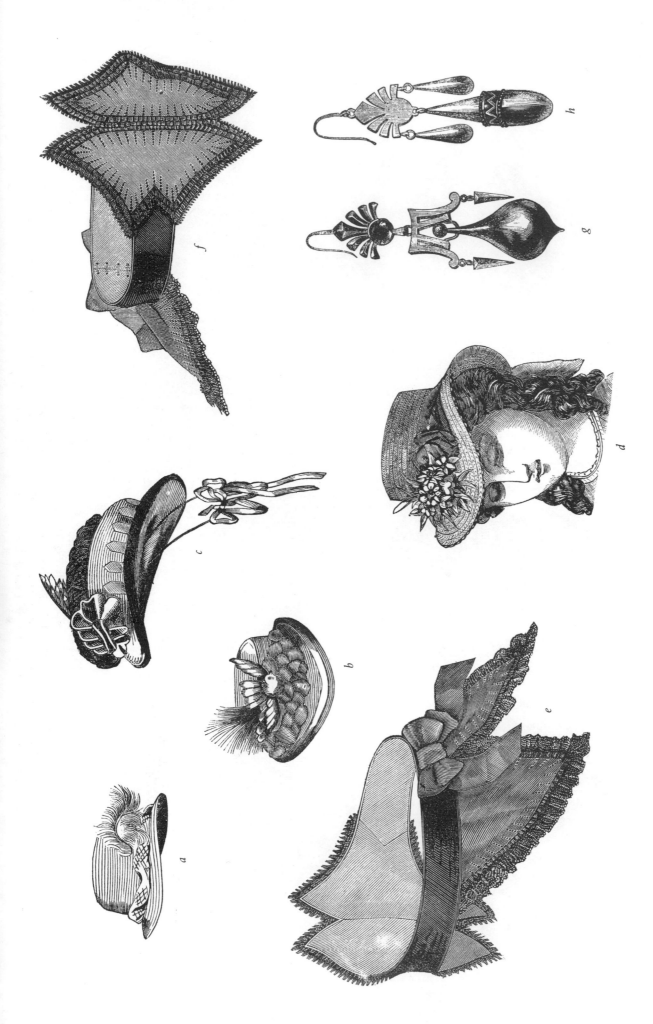

Fig. a: Hat of *paille de riz*; edge bound with cerise velvet; plaid ribbon and large ostrich feather on left side. *Fig. b:* White straw hat bound with scarlet velvet and trimmed with white marabout feathers, a scarlet bird and an aigrette of spun glass. *Fig. c:* Black and white straw hat with blue and green velvet and peacock feathers (7/65). *Fig. d:* White straw hat trimmed with scarlet velvet and bunch of white flowers and green leaves (5/65). *Figs. e & f:* Front and back views of the "Marguerite" girdle. The band is of black velvet; the plastron in front and basque of any contrasting color; trimmings, fluted black lace and still beads; band laces at back under bow (1/65). *Fig. g:* Earring of dead gold; pendant of rock crystal. *Fig. h:* Earring of gold and coral, clasped in a fancy band of enamel (9/65).

EVENING DRESSES. *Fig. a:* Dress of light sea-green silk trimmed with bands of straw worked with black; front of dress is formed of Cluny lace and bands of straw. *Fig. b:* Petticoat of blue silk trimmed with tarlatan ruffles; overdress of tarlatan or crape. *Fig. c:* Dress of white silk trimmed with quillings of pink silk or crape; rosettes of ribbon or velvet (7/67).

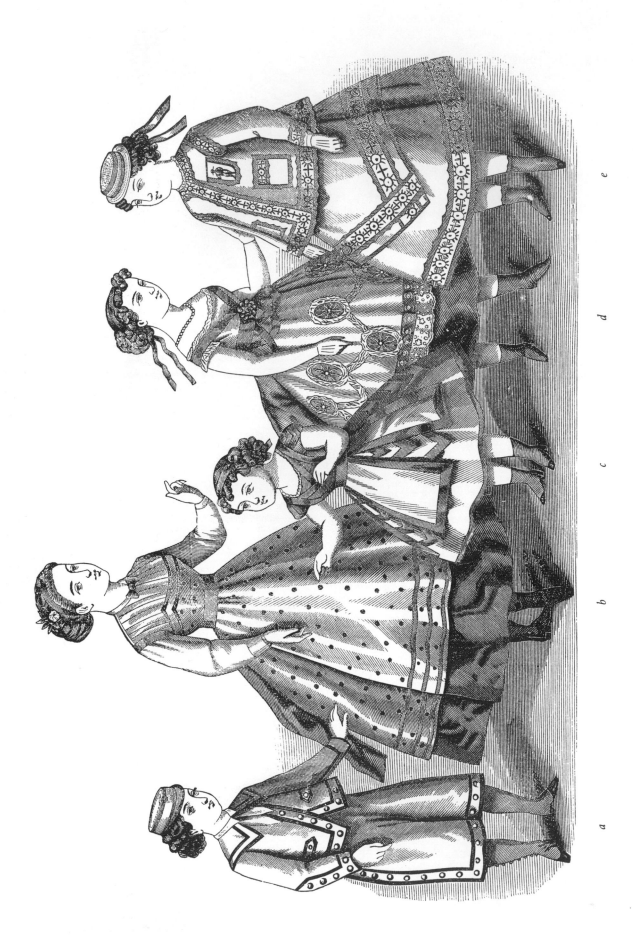

CHILDREN'S DRESSES. *Fig. a:* Suit for a little boy, of buff piqué trimmed with black mohair braid and jet buttons; straw cap with black velvet trim. *Fig. b:* Underskirt of blue silk; overdress of *satin de mair* of white ground with large satin balls; trimming of blue satin. *Fig. c:* Dress of white piqué trimmed with bias bands of blue cambric. *Fig. d:* Underskirt of rose-colored silk; overdress of blue French muslin finished with Cluny lace headed by an insertion of rose-colored ribbon. *Fig. e:* Suit of white mohair ornamented with bands of braiding in black, finished with a row of green velvet; hat is white chip and green velvet (8/67).

76

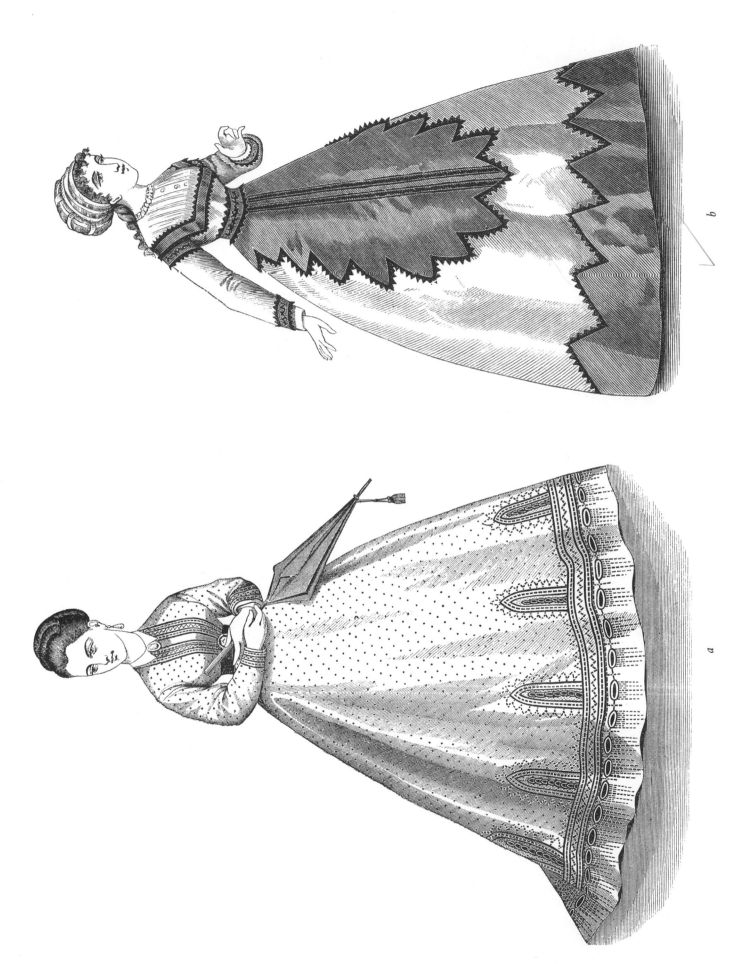

Fig. a: Robe dress of white percale dotted in dark blue; border in black and blue (8/67). *Fig. b:* Dinner dress of pearl-colored silk trimmed with magenta silk edged with black lace (11/67).

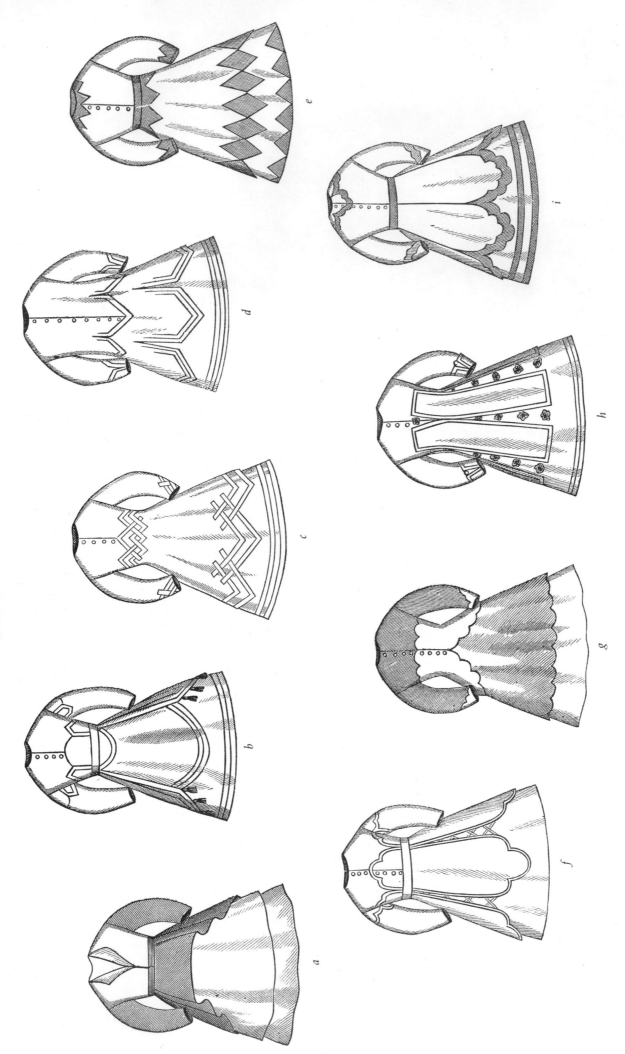

FALL STYLES FOR CHILDREN. *Fig. a*: Dress of gray cashmere with peplum of scarlet cashmere. *Fig. b*: Dress for little boy, of piqué, merino or alpaca; trimming of velvet or braid. *Fig. c*: Boy's dress of Bismarck poplin trimmed with straps of bronzed leather. *Fig. d*: Suit of blue silk trimmed with bands of blue velvet. *Fig. e*: Girl's dress of white cashmere trimmed with rose-silk diamonds and border. *Fig. f*: Dress, suitable for boy or girl, of bright blue merino trimmed with black-and-white braid. *Fig. g*: Girl's dress; upper part of green poplin; lower part of gray. *Fig. h*: Little girl's costume of rose velvet merino trimmed with narrow velvet and rosettes of rose-colored silk. *Fig. i*: Dress of brown poplin trimmed with darker shade; this model would answer for a walking dress for a little boy or girl (10/67).

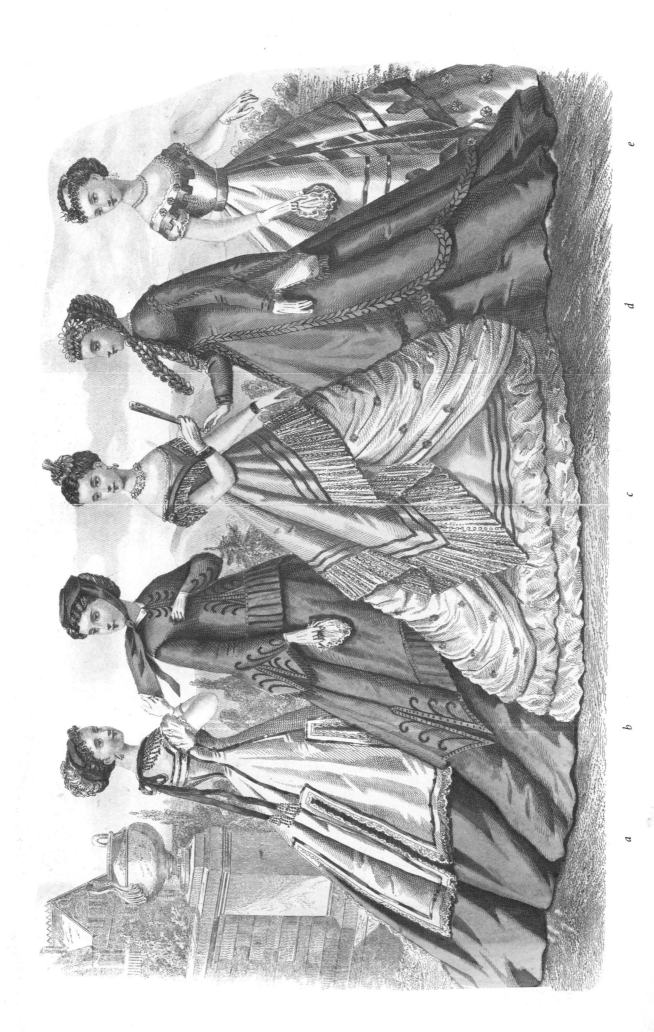

Fig. a: Evening dress of pink silk with overdress of white silk trimmed with pink; dress is gored *à l'Impératrice* or body and skirt cut in one. *Fig. b:* Walking suit of Bismarck silk trimmed with applications of black velvet; bonnet of purple silk. *Fig. c:* Evening dress of green silk trimmed with bands of darker velvet and white crape lisse; skirt of white crape lisse starred with gold draped over skirt of green with puffed white crape at hem. *Fig. d:* Visiting dress of purple silk. *Fig. e:* Dress for a young lady, of white silk trimmed with blue (9/67).

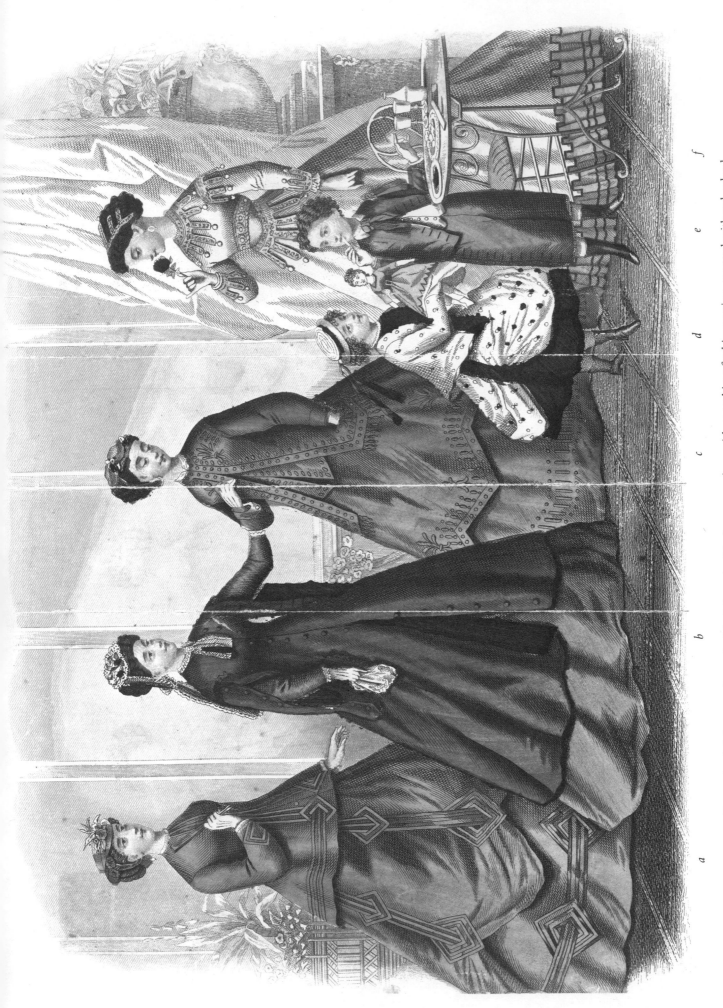

Fig. a: Walking suit of violet reps trimmed with violet satin. *Fig. b:* Morning costume; redingote or overdress of black silk with a scarlet quilted lining; underskirt and sleeves of green poplin. *Fig. c:* Visiting dress of Bismarck silk. *Fig. d:* Little girl's dress of scarlet merino, with overskirt of white merino, spotted with red, edged with black. *Fig. e:* Little boy's suit of fine brown cloth. *Fig. f:* Dinner dress of pearl-colored silk trimmed with luminous green silk (11/67).

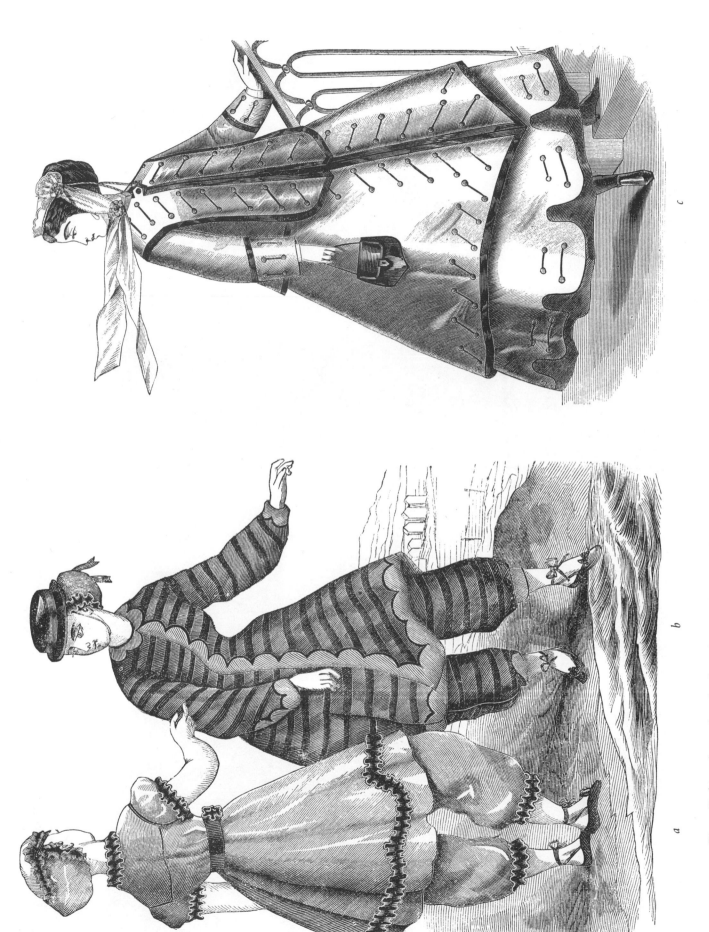

Fig. a: Bathing dress of scarlet flannel trimmed with plaiting of black flannel bound with white braid; cap of oil-silk trimmed with scarlet and black. *Fig. b:* Bathing dress of scarlet and black bathing cloth; paletot turned up with scarlet flannel cut in scallops edged with black braid; hat is of black glazed cloth trimmed with scarlet (7/65). *Fig. c:* Promenade suit of purple velvet, purple cord and velvet buttons (12/67).

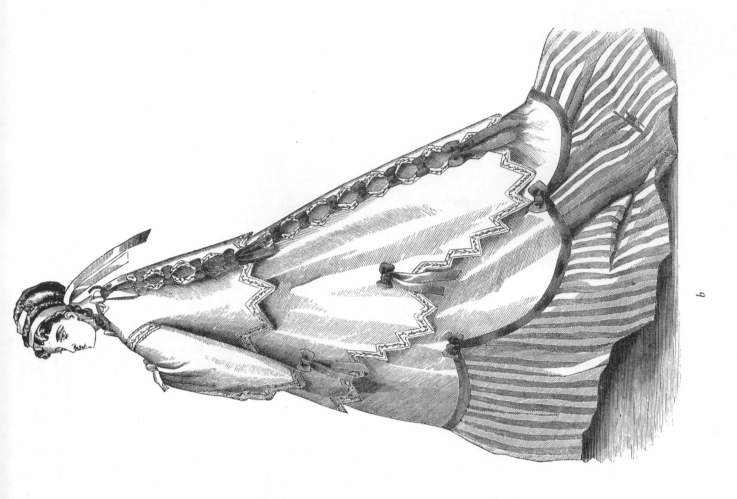

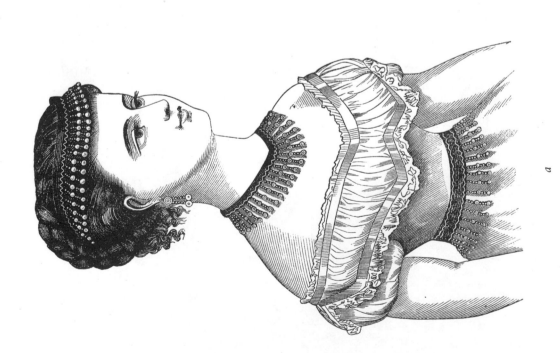

Fig. a: The "May bell ornaments"; bandelet around the head, the necklet and trimming below waistband are of small straw bells and crystal beads. These are attached to black velvet ribbons (8/67).

Fig. b: Morning robe; underskirt of white alpaca with flounce of blue-and-white-striped silk; bound with blue ribbon; overdress of white alpaca trimmed with Cluny inserting lined with blue (9/67).

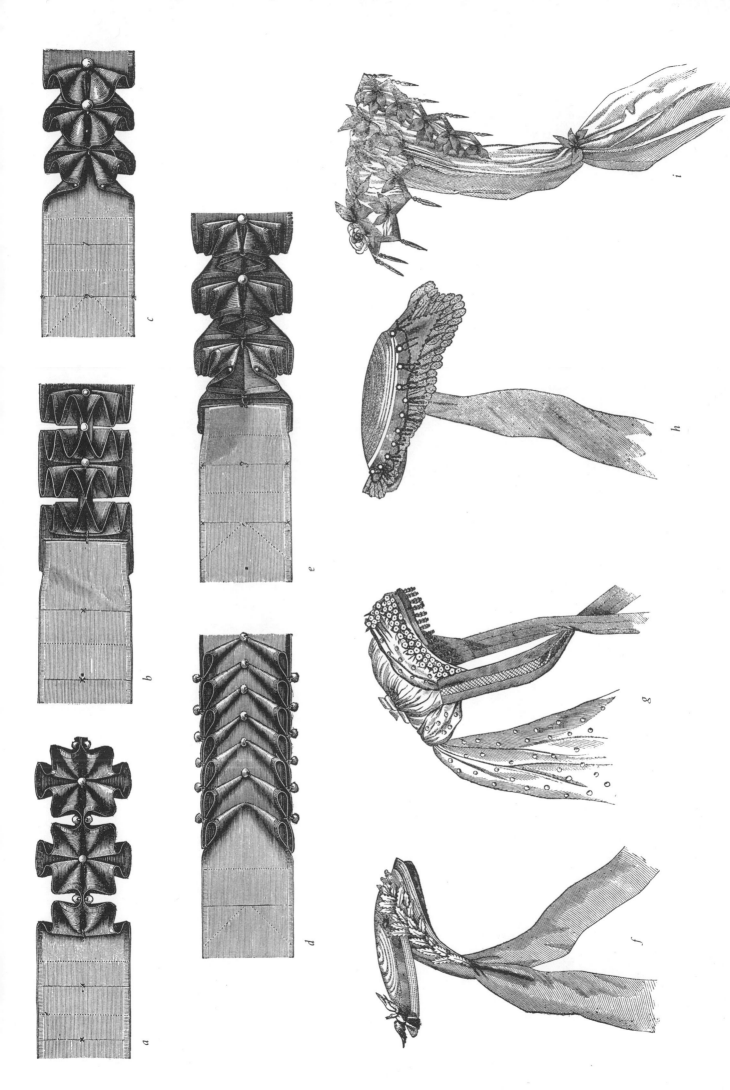

Figs. a–e: Ribbon trimmings (10/67). *Fig. f:* Straw bonnet trimmed with oak leaves, bird of gay plumage and green silk ribbons. *Fig. g:* Bonnet of white tulle with fringe of crystal drops and small white flowers; scarf of beaded tulle (8/67). *Fig. h:* Hat of white straw trimmed with blue velvet edged with black lace and crystal beads. *Fig. i:* Bonnet of white tulle, made on a frame pointed on all the edges; points bound in green velvet; the whole covered with tufts of green leaves (9/67).

83

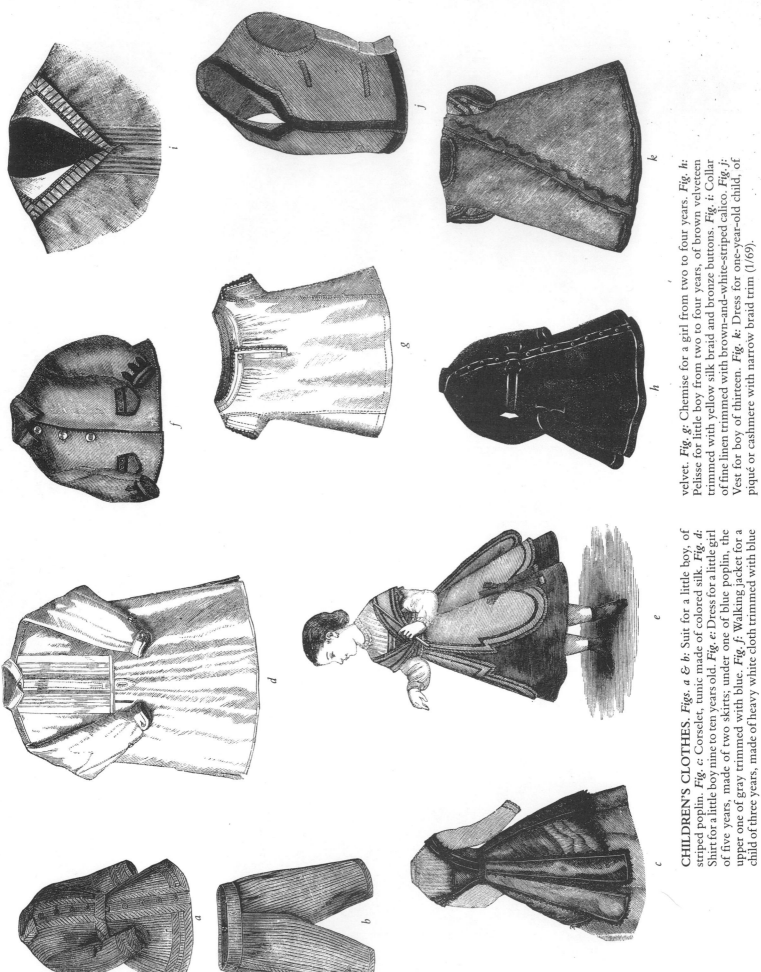

CHILDREN'S CLOTHES. *Figs. a & b:* Suit for a little boy, of striped poplin. *Fig. c:* Corselet, tunic made of colored silk. *Fig. d:* Shirt for a little boy nine to ten years old. *Fig. e:* Dress for a little girl of five years, made of two skirts; under one of blue poplin, the upper one of gray trimmed with blue. *Fig. f:* Walking jacket for a child of three years, made of heavy white cloth trimmed with blue

velvet. *Fig. g:* Chemise for a girl from two to four years. *Fig. h:* Pelisse for little boy from two to four years, of brown velveteen trimmed with yellow silk braid and bronze buttons. *Fig. i:* Collar of fine linen trimmed with brown-and-white-striped calico. *Fig. j:* Vest for boy of thirteen. *Fig. k:* Dress for one-year-old child, of piqué or cashmere with narrow braid trim (1/69).

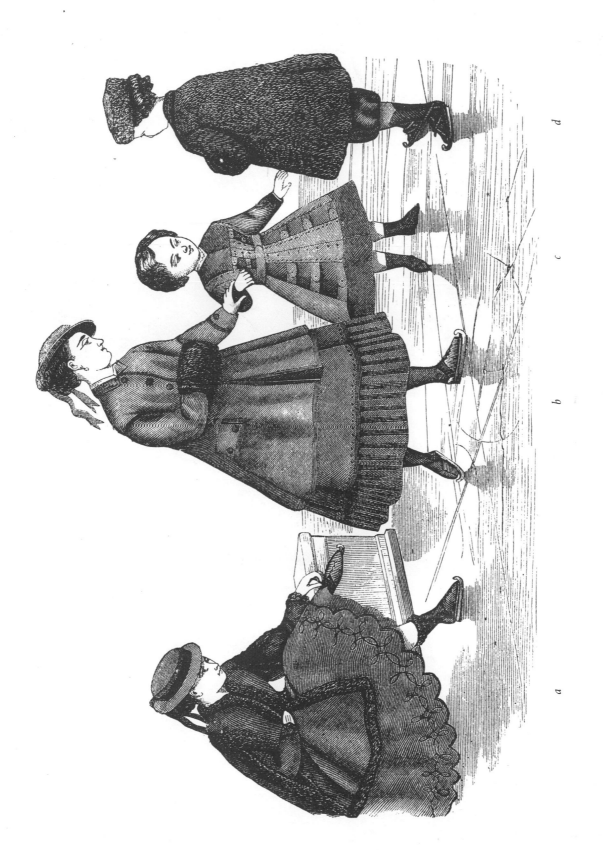

SKATING COSTUMES FOR CHILDREN. *Fig. a:* Dress and coat of blue poplin; coat trimmed with fur; hat of glazed leather. *Fig. b:* Dress and underskirt of scarlet poplin. *Fig. c:* Little boy's dress of crimson merino; overdress of stone color. *Fig. d:* Boy's costume; Garibaldi pants of black velvet; sacque of Astrakhan cloth (1/69).

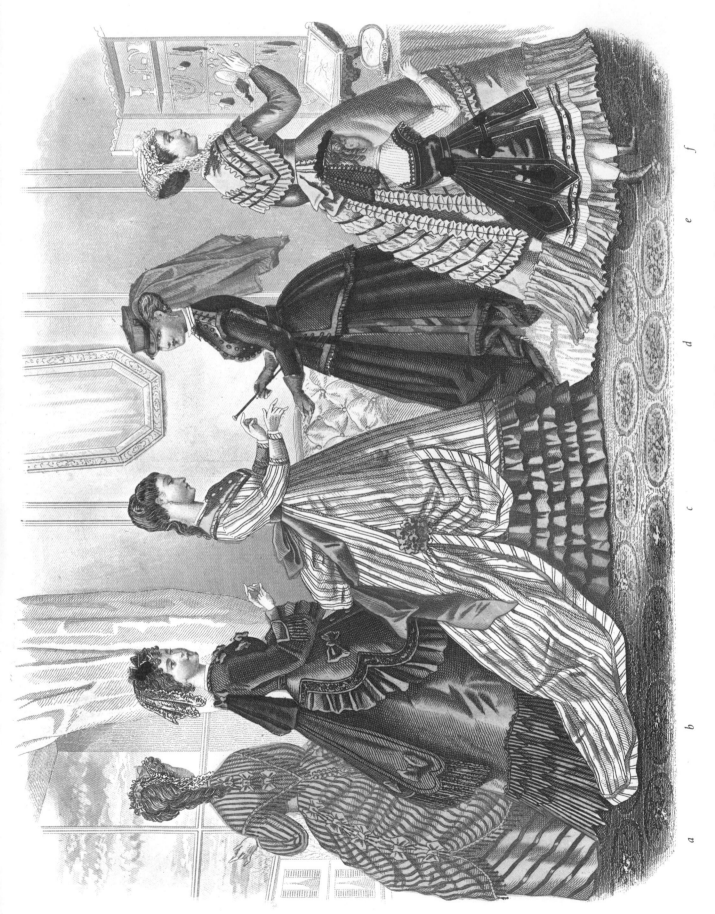

Fig. a: Walking dress of blue-and-black-striped silk. *Fig. b:* Walking suit of Havana-brown poplin. *Fig. c:* Dinner dress of green-and-white-striped silk trimmed with green silk. *Fig. d:* Riding habit of fine black cloth bound with cuir-colored poplin. *Fig. e:* Walking dress of lilac silk poplin; white crape bonnet. *Fig. f:* Dress for little girl, of black and white silk; overdress of black silk with cherry-colored rosettes (4/69).

a   b   c   d   e   f

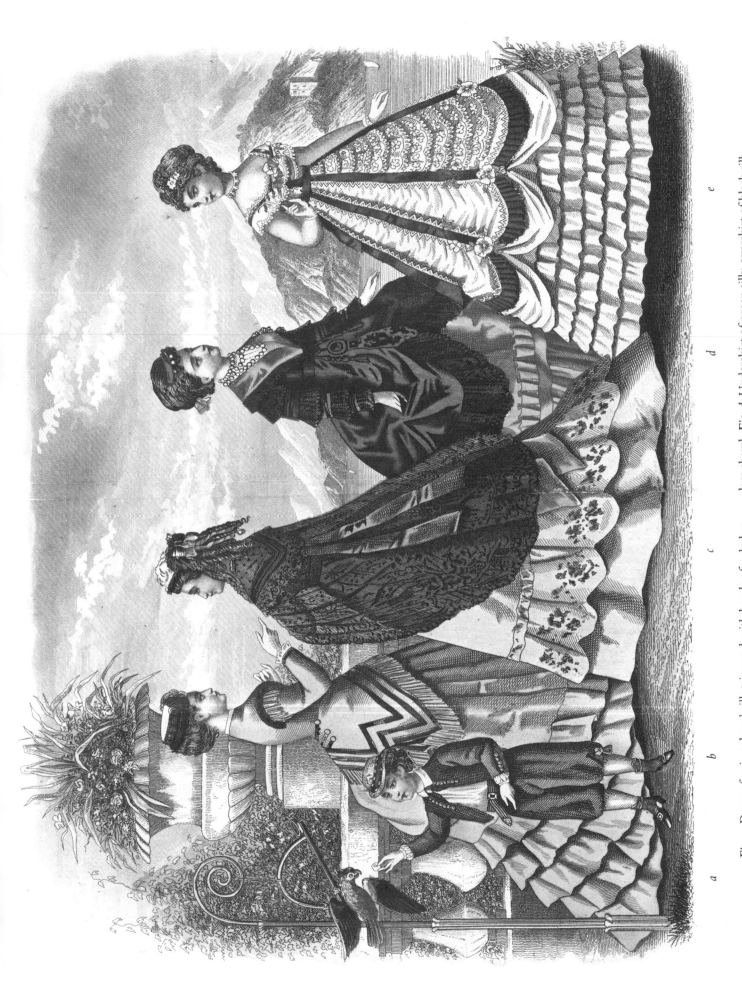

Fig. a: Dress of cuir-colored silk trimmed with bands of a darker color; white chip straw hat. *Fig. b:* Boy's costume; purple cloth made in Zouave style; Garibaldi pants; gray stockings and purple boots. *Fig. c:* Robe of lilac grenadine; sash of purple ribbon; black

lace shawl. *Fig. d:* Underskirt of green silk; overskirt of black silk trimmed with lace. *Fig. e:* Evening dress of white muslin with deep-rose ribbon trim (6/69).

87

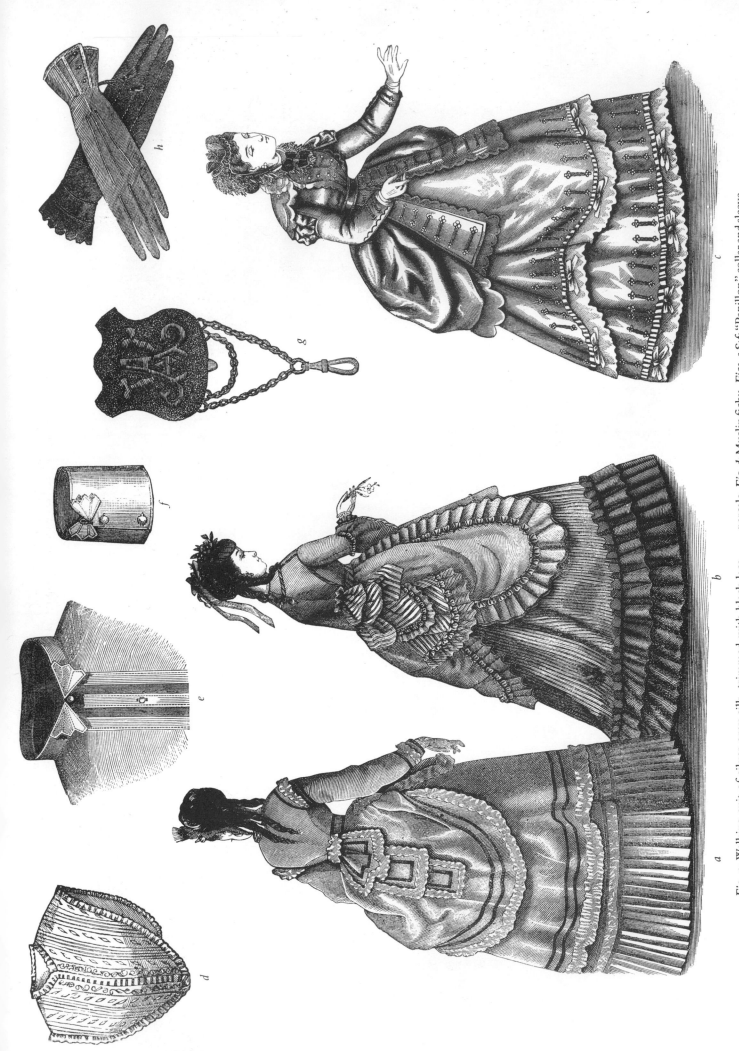

Fig. a: Walking suit of silver-gray silk, trimmed with black lace (7/69). Fig. b: Dress of pale green silk. Fig. c: Suit; underskirt of blue and striped percale with blue ruffles; upper skirt and waist of blue

percale. Fig. d: Muslin fichu. Figs. e & f: "Papillon" collar and sleeve of white linen. Fig. g: Chatelaine ornament for keys, fan, etc. Fig. h: Kid gloves (8/69).

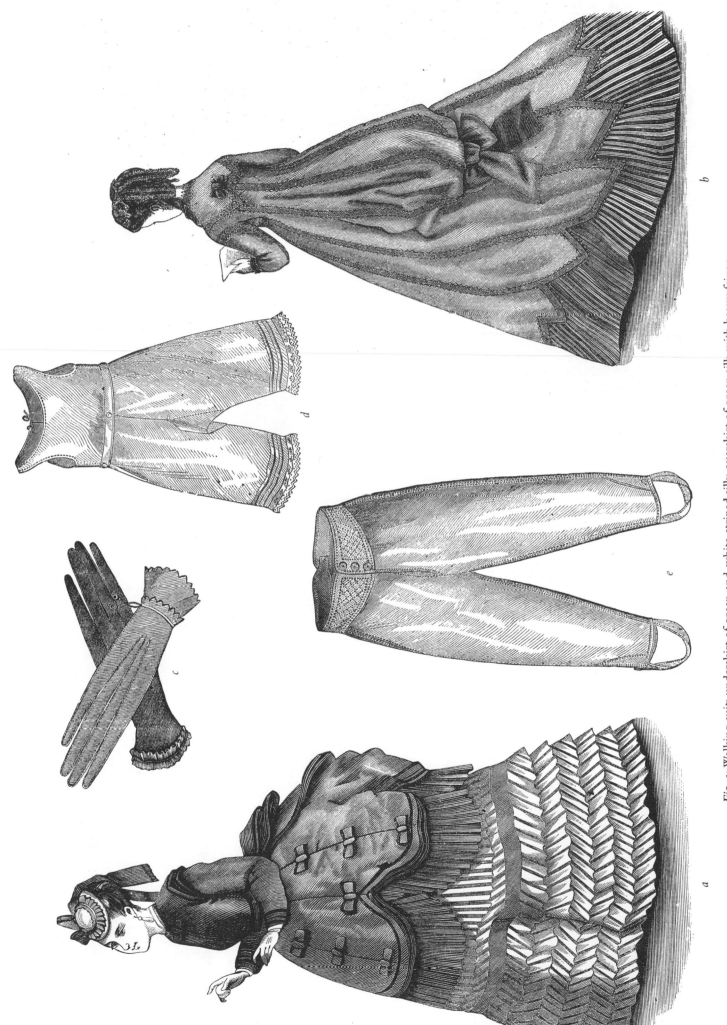

Fig. a: Walking suit; underskirt of green-and-white-striped silk; overskirt of green silk with heavy fringe. *Fig. b:* Morning robe. *Fig. c:* Kid gloves. *Fig. d:* Bodice and drawers for little boy of three or four years. *Fig. e:* Gentleman's drawers (9/69).

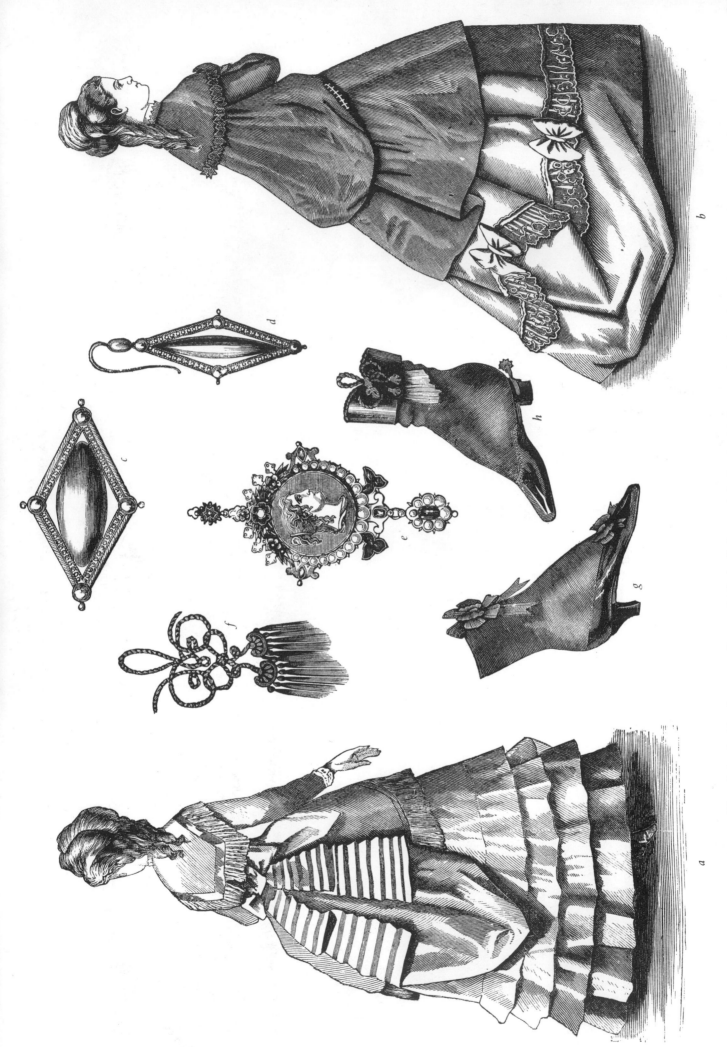

Fig. a: Suit of golden-brown poplin. *Fig. b*: Black silk dress and cloak. *Figs. c & d*: Roman brooch and earring.
Fig. e: Cameo pendant framed in gold. *Fig. f*: Gimp tassel. *Fig. g*: Kid boot trimmed with ribbon. *Fig. h*:
Riding boot of kid with patent-leather tops (11/69).

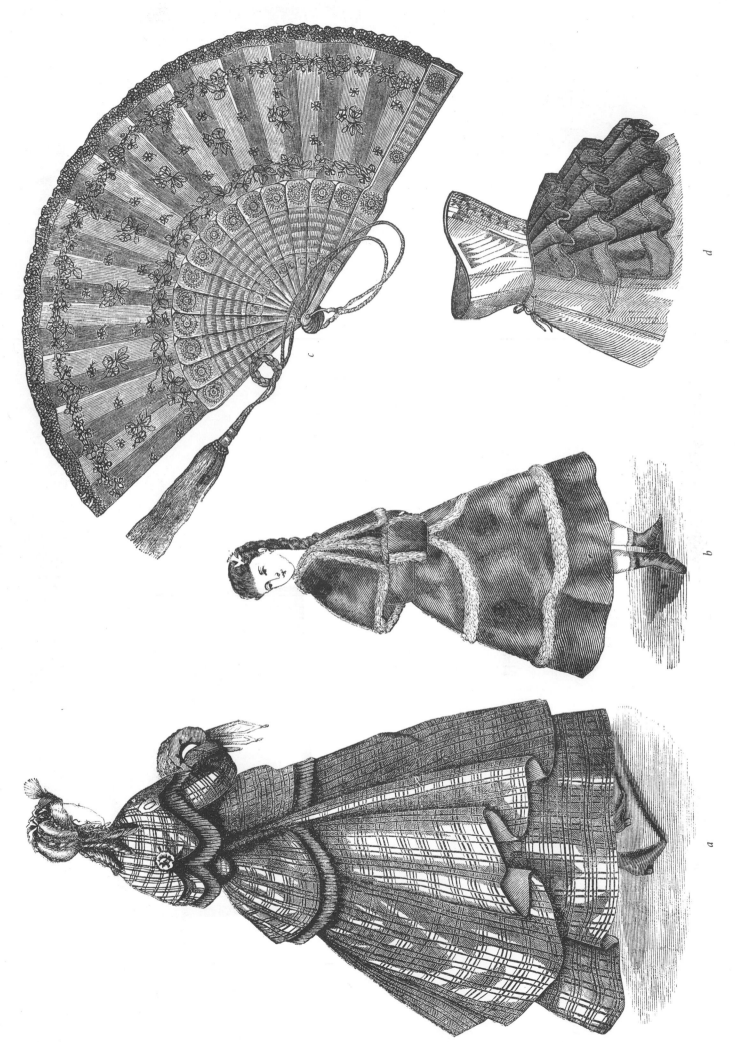

Fig. a: Suit of green-and-blue-plaid poplin. *Fig. b*: Suit for a girl of twelve years, made of blue velvet trimmed with fur (12/69). *Fig. c*: Fan of patterned ivory covered with white *glacé* silk and embroidered in fine black silk (1/69). *Fig. d*: Horsehair pannier to wear with puffed dresses (4/69).